EMERGENCY NURSING PROCEDURES

POCKET MANUAL SERIES™

Pocket Manual of

EMERGENCY NURSING PROCEDURES

MARY E. MANCINI, RN, MSN, CNA

Vice-President, Nursing Administration
Parkland Memorial Hospital
Dallas, Texas

1988
B.C. Decker Inc • Toronto • Philadelphia

Publisher

B.C. Decker Inc
3228 South Service Road
Burlington, Ontario   L7N 3H8

B.C. Decker Inc
320 Walnut Street
Suite 400
Philadelphia, Pennsylvania   19106

Sales and Distribution

United States and Possessions	**The C.V. Mosby Company** 11830 Westline Industrial Drive Saint Louis, Missouri 63146
Canada	**The C.V. Mosby Company, Ltd.** 5240 Finch Avenue East, Unit No. 1 Scarborough, Ontario M1S 5P2
United Kingdom, Europe and the Middle East	**Blackwell Scientific Publications, Ltd.** Osney Mead, Oxford OX2 OEL, England
Australia and New Zealand	**Harcourt Brace Jovanovich Group** **(Australia) Pty Limited** 30–52 Smidmore Street Marrickville, N.S.W. 2204 Australia
Japan	**Igaku-Shoin Ltd.** Tokyo International P.O. Box 5063 1–28–36 Hongo, Bunkyo-ku, Tokyo 113, Japan
Asia	**Info-Med Ltd.** 802–3 Ruttonjee House 11 Duddell Street Central Hong Kong
South Africa	**Libriger Book Distributors** Warehouse Number 8 "Die Ou Looiery" Tannery Road Hamilton, Bloemfontein 9300
South America	**Inter-Book Marketing Services** Rua das Palmeriras, 32 Apto. 701 222–70 Rio de Janeiro RJ, Brazil

Pocket Manual of Emergency Nursing Procedures   ISBN 1-55664-068-4

Library of Congress catalog card number: 87-73453

10 9 8 7 6 5 4 3 2 1

To David and Laura

CONTRIBUTORS

JERRY BROCK, RN

Head Nurse, Inpatient Psychiatry, Parkland Memorial Hospital, Dallas, Texas

CARLA CALLOWAY, RN, BSN, CCRN

Patient Educator, Parkland Memorial Hospital, Dallas, Texas

PAMELA Y. DONNELLY, RN, MSN

Staff Nurse, Labor and Delivery, Parkland Memorial Hospital, Dallas, Texas

KATHY GILLILAND, RN, BSN

Spinal Cord Specialist, Parkland Memorial Hospital, Dallas, Texas

JOY A. GORZEMAN, RN, MSN

Nursing Education Coordinator, Parkland Memorial Hospital, Dallas, Texas

LISA A. JONES, RN, BSN, CEN

Head Nurse, Emergency Services, Parkland Memorial Hospital, Dallas, Texas

BARBARA KALO, RNC, BSN

Nurse Educator, Parkland Memorial Hospital, Dallas, Texas

KAREN KRENTZ, RN, BSN

Emergency Services Nurse Educator, Parkland Memorial Hospital, Dallas, Texas

LAURA LUECKE, RN, BSN, CCRN

Nurse Educator, Parkland Memorial Hospital, Dallas, Texas

MARY E. MANCINI, RN, MSN, CNA

Vice-President, Nursing Administration, Parkland Memorial Hospital, Dallas, Texas

JEAN MASON, RN, BSN, MPA

Assistant Director, Emergency Services, Parkland Memorial Hospital, Dallas, Texas

BARBARA CLARK MIMS, RN, MSN, CCRN

Nurse Internship Coordinator, Parkland Memorial Hospital, Dallas, Texas

LISA MORRA-MARTIN, RN, BSN, CCRN

Nurse Internship Instructor, Parkland Memorial Hospital, Dallas, Texas

PAULA K. OVENS, RN, MS

Nurse Recruiter, Parkland Memorial Hospital,
Dallas, Texas

JORIE SCOTT, RN

Trauma Coordinator, Parkland Memorial Hospital,
Dallas, Texas

MOLLY A. SEAMAN, RN, MSN, CEN

Administrative Assistant, Emergency Services, Parkland
Memorial Hospital, Dallas, Texas

ROBERT STEELE, RN, BSN, CCRN

Staff Nurse, Emergency Services, Parkland Memorial
Hospital, Dallas, Texas

KATHLEEN H. TOTO, RN, BSN, CCRN

Nurse Internship Instructor, Parkland Memorial Hospital,
Dallas, Texas

NANCY WEINBERG, RN

Nurse Recruiter, Parkland Memorial Hospital,
Dallas, Texas

LINDA WELD, RN, MSN

Critical Care Coordinator, Parkland Memorial Hospital,
Dallas, Texas

CONTENTS

I

EMERGENCY PROCEDURES

RESPIRATORY PROCEDURES

OBSTETRICAL AND GYNECOLOGIC PROCEDURES

EYE, EAR, NOSE, AND THROAT PROCEDURES

VASCULAR PROCEDURES

DIAGNOSTIC PROCEDURES

OTHER PROCEDURES

II

ASSESSMENT GUIDELINES

III

APPENDICES

INTRODUCTION

The *Pocket Manual of Emergency Nursing Procedures* was developed to provide Emergency Department nurses with a quick reference to a variety of procedures that they frequently encounter. These procedures are presented in a format most useful to the nurse: in an easily readable listing, the book provides the purpose, indications, contraindications, equipment, step-by-step procedures, follow-up, and documentation for each included procedure. Each procedure is structured in a manner amenable for use as a standard of care or quality assurance monitor.

Four assessment guidelines are included. Cardiac, neurologic, respiratory, and trauma assessments are outlined. These step-by-step guidelines can be used as a ready reference when emergency patients arrive.

The appendices include the 1987 American Heart Association Algorithms for Advanced Cardiac Life Support. Additionally, listings of blood products, isolation procedures, intravenous medication administration, and normals for the most common laboratory tests are provided. It should be noted that standards given in these appendices are specific to Parkland Memorial Hospital and may vary somewhat from institution to institution.

I would also like to thank Jan Coder, Senior Administrative Assistant, and Kathy Grey, Medical Illustrator, for their invaluable assistance in the preparation of this book.

I

EMERGENCY PROCEDURES

RESPIRATORY PROCEDURES

1

CRICOTHYROIDOTOMY

JORIE SCOTT

Purpose

To provide safe, fast, emergent surgical airway management

Indications

- Medical emergencies that occlude the airway–
    - epiglottitis
    - acute peritonsillar abscess
    - postsurgical complications
    - associated facial trauma
- Questionable unstable neck injury when nasotracheal intubation cannot be readily achieved

Contraindications

- Not recommended in pediatric patients under 12 years. (Note: there is a 40–50% incidence of a pneumothorax developing after a surgical airway procedure.)
- Injury to trachea when landmarks are not easily identified

Potential Complications

- Tracheal stenosis
- Bleeding that may be difficult to control

- Asphyxia
- Aspiration
- Cellulitis
- Esophageal perforation
- Exsanguinating hematoma
- Tracheal posterior wall perforation
- Thyroid perforation
- Inadequate ventilation leading to hypoxia or death
- Laryngeal stenosis
- Laceration of esophagus
- Vocal cord paralysis
- Hoarseness

Equipment

Betadine
4 × 4 gauze sponges
Gauze packing
#12 to #14 gauge over-the-needle catheter
Jet insufflation equipment:
  Y-connector and oxygen tubing
  Wall mounted oxygen or oxygen tank with flow meter
Syringe (5 or 10 ml)
Hemostats
Tracheostomy tube #4, #5
3.0-mm endotracheal (ET) tube
Lidocaine (without epinephrine) 10 ml
Twill tape
Retractors, tracheal hook, tracheal spreader
Mask, gloves, gown
Electrocautery
Light source
Determine if *Needle Cricothyroidomtomy* is to be attempted first or
go directly to *Surgical Cricothyroidotomy*.

Needle Cricothyroidotomy

Procedure

1. Assess patient's airway, breathing, and circulation (ABCs), and intervene to protect and provide a patent airway
2. Notify physician of possible airway compromise
3. Assess for respiratory adequacy; foreign body in oral cavity
4. Obtain arterial blood gases
5. Assemble equipment, plug in electrocautery
6. Administer sedation if necessary
7. Place patient in a supine position with neck in alignment
8. Assist physician in preparing the area
9. Direct light source to neck area
10. Assist physician with gloves, gown, and mask
11. Assist physician in establishing sterile field
12. Open over-the-needle catheter onto sterile field
13. Open 3.0-mm pediatric endotracheal tube onto sterile field
14. Connect Y-connector to oxygen tubing to flow meter at 15 L/min (50 psi)
15. Assist physician as the needle is inserted at a 45 degree angle into the lower half of the cricothyroid membrane (Fig. 1–1)
16. Observe for aspiration of air
17. Assist in controlling bleeding as indicated
18. Assess lung expansion by auscultation
19. Secure apparatus to neck

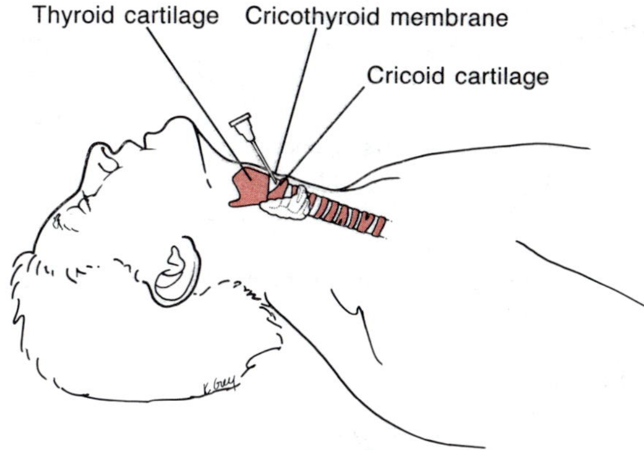

Figure 1–1 Anatomical landmarks for needle cricothyroidotomy.

Surgical Cricothyroidotomy

Procedure

Steps 1 through 11 are the same as for the needle cricothyroid-otomy procedure

12. If patient conscious, assist physician in anesthetizing local area
13. Open ET or tracheostomy tube as indicated onto sterile field
14. Assist respiratory therapist in setting up ventilator, or supplemental oxygen with adaptors as indicated
15. Assist physician by directing light onto neck, maintain neck in neutral position, have syringe ready to inflate tracheosto-my cuff
16. Assist in controlling bleeding as indicated
17. Observe chest expansion after cuff is inflated
18. Auscultate chest bilaterally for adequate ventilation
19. Assist physician in securing tube

Follow-Up

1. Assist respiratory therapist in assuring adequate ventilation
2. Reassess patient's ABCs
3. Obtain repeat arterial blood gases
4. Continue to monitor and document vital signs and level of consciousness q15min as indicated
5. Assist with ongoing emergent interventions
6. Alert Operating Room if patient needs further surgical intervention

Documentation

Initial assessment of patient
Procedure used and outcome
Ongoing respiratory assessment

SUGGESTED READING

American College of Surgeons Committee on Trauma. Advanced trauma life support. Chicago: American College of Surgeons, 1985:23–40.

Boyd AD. A clinical evaluation of cricothyroidotomy. Surg Gynecol Obstet 1979; 149:365.

Eckstein K. Nursing process in multiple trauma. In: Holloway NM. Emergency Department Nurses Association. Core curriculum. Philadelphia: WB Saunders, 1985:239.

2

ENDOTRACHEAL INTUBATION
BARBARA CLARK MIMS

Purpose
To establish a patent airway

Indications
- Need for mechanical ventilation
- Need for pulmonary hygiene
- Potential aspiration
- Potential upper airway obstruction
- Administration of anesthesia

Contraindications
- No absolute contraindications; however, severe upper airway edema or fractures of the face and neck may make intubation impossible

Potential Complications
- Bruises, lacerations, and abrasions
- Nosebleed (with nasotracheal intubation)
- Airway obstruction (herniation of cuff, kinking of tube)
- Sinusitis (with nasotracheal tube)
- Tracheal rupture
- Tracheoesophageal fistula

- Vomiting with aspiration
- Tooth loss or damage
- Cardiac dysrhythmias

Equipment

Endotracheal (ET) tubes of various sizes
Stylet
Laryngoscope, curved and straight blades
MacGill forceps (for nasotracheal intubation only)
Anesthetic jelly
4 × 4 gauze sponges
Syringe (10 ml)
Oral pharyngeal airway
Resuscitation bag with adapter and mask connected to oxygen tub-
   ing and flowmeter
Suction apparatus
Suction catheter with sterile glove
Yankauer tonsil suction tip
1-inch adhesive tape
Cardiac arrest cart
Ventilator or oxygen setup as ordered
Wrist restraints
Cardiac monitor or electrocardiograph machine

Procedure

1. Notify respiratory therapist, and obtain ventilator or oxygen setup as ordered by the physician
2. Explain procedure to patient, if feasible. Restrain as necessary.
3. Assure that patient has a patent intravenous line
4. Position cardiac arrest cart at bedside

5. Check to be sure suction equipment and ambu bag are set up and functioning. Attach Yankauer suction tip to suction source.
6. If patient is not on a cardiac monitor, connect either to a monitor or to an electrocardiograph machine
7. Remove head of bed or stretcher and position patient as close to the head of bed or stretcher as possbile. The patient should be positioned in the *sniffing position*, in which the neck is flexed with the head extended. This may be achieved by placing 2 to 4 inches of firm padding underneath head.
8. Ask physician which type of blade is preferred and what size ET tube is to be used
9. Attach blade to laryngoscope, and check bulb for proper illumination
10. Obtain ET tube, and inflate cuff to check for symmetrical expansion and leaks
11. Lubricate distal half of ET tube with anesthetic jelly
12. Insert stylet into tube, making sure it does not protrude beyond tip of ET tube
13. Be prepared to administer intravenous drugs (succinylcholine or diazepam)
14. Hand the lubricated ET tube with universal adapter and stylet in place, laryngoscope with blade attached, and oral pharyngeal airway to the physician
15. Observe and support patient. Keep intravenous line patent, and watch for dysrhythmias
16. Apply cricoid pressure during endotracheal intubation to protect against regurgitation of gastric contents. Find cricoid cartilage by first palpating depression just below thyroid cartilage (Adam's apple). The prominence inferior to this cartilage is the cricoid cartilage. Apply pressure to anterolateral aspects of the cartilage just lateral to the midline, using thumb and index finger. Maintain pressure until cuff on the endotracheal tube has been inflated (Fig. 2-1).

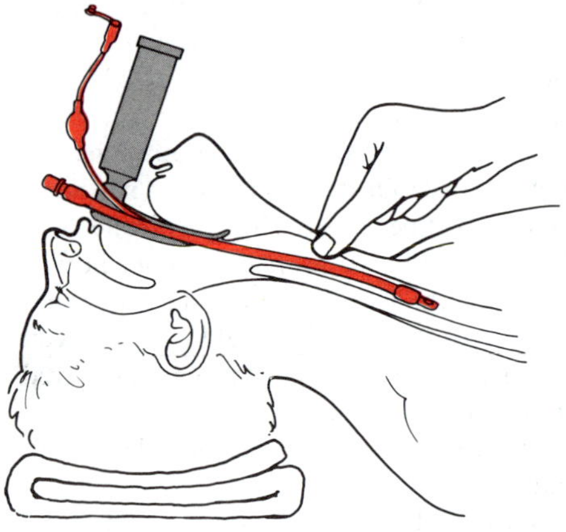

Figure 2–1 Applying cricoid pressure until cuff is inflated during endotracheal intubation.

17. Once ET tube is in place, inflate cuff with minimal occlusive volume as follows:
    a) During inspiration (manual resuscitation bag or ventilator), slowly inject air into cuff filling line. Withhold cuff inflation during expiratory cycle.
    b) Resume slow cuff inflation during the subsequent inspiratory cycle
    c) Terminate cuff inflation when leakage just stops
18. Suction and ventilate as indicated
19. To check ET tube position, ventilate with bag and auscultate breath sounds. Observe for bilateral chest excursions.
20. Secure ET tube in place as follows:
    a) For orally intubated patients who are not edentulous, insert oral pharyngeal airway or bite block between teeth. (If oral pharyngeal airway is used, it should be cut off so that it does not extend into posterior pharynx.)

b) Tear two pieces of 1-inch adhesive tape, one approximately 20–24 inches long and the other approximately 14–16 inches long (enough to go around the patient's head and wrap around the ET tube several times)

c) Place the 20- to 24-inch strip on a flat surface, sticky side up, and back the tape with the 14- to 16-inch strip

d) Apply benzoin to skin at sides of mouth

e) Place tape behind patient's neck

f) Split each end of tape lengthwise for a distance of 4–5 inches

g) Place one tail of one piece of tape across the mouth above the lips, then wind the other tail around the ET tube at the point where it enters the mouth

h) Place one tail of the other end of the tape below the lower lip across the chin, then wind the other tail around the ET tube at the point where the tube enters the mouth

i) Auscultate chest for bilateral breath sounds

Follow-Up

1. Ensure that ET tube is secure and that patient is ventilating adequately
2. Assess oxygen device or ventilator
3. Order stat portable chest x-ray film to check ET tube placement
4. Reassure and comfort patient

Documentation

Size of ET tube and route of insertion
Amount of air required to establish minimal occlusive volume
Patient's tolerance of procedure

SUGGESTED READING

Millar S, Sampson LK, Soukup M. AACN Procedure manual for critical care. Philadelphia: WB Saunders, 1985:210.

Persons CB. Critical care procedures and protocols. A nursing process approach. Philadelphia: JB Lippincott, 1987:247.

Shaprio BA, Harrison RA, Trout CA. Clinical application of respiratory care. Chicago: Year Book Medical Publishers, 1979:242, 281.

Smith S, Duell D. Clinical nursing skills. Los Altos: National Nursing Review, 1985:670.

3

ESOPHAGEAL OBTURATOR AIRWAY INSERTION

MOLLY A. SEAMAN

Purpose

To provide a patent airway and ventilation for the apneic unconscious patient

Indications

- Respiratory arrest
- Cardiac arrest

Contraindications

- Children under 16 years of age
- Conscious or semiconscious adults
- Patients with suspected foreign bodies of trachea, ingestion of corrosive chemicals, or esophageal disease

Potential Complications

- Tracheal intubation
- Esophageal injury
- Vomiting

Equipment

Esophageal obturator airway (EOA) tube and mask
Syringe (30–35 ml)

Wall suction or suction machine and suction catheter or tip
Bag-valve-mask device
Lubricant (water-soluble)

Procedure

1. Maintain artificial ventilation until EOA tube is available
2. Before insertion of tube, test balloon on cuff for any leaks
3. Lie patient in a supine position, and pull mandible straight upward
4. With other hand, insert lubricated EOA tube into patient's mouth. Curvature of tube should follow same natural curvature of pharynx. Never use force during insertion of tube. If obstruction is felt, withdraw tube slightly, improve tongue-jaw lift and readvance tube (Fig. 3–1).

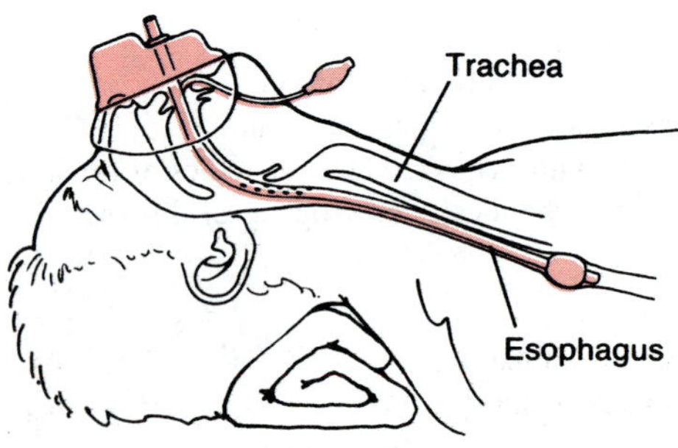

Figure 3–1 Correct placement of esophageal obturator airway.

5. Gently advance tube until mask is sealed on patient's face
6. With mask firmly sealed to face, check position of EOA tube. Use bag-valve device to blow into tube. Tube is correctly placed when chest rises with ventilation.
7. If chest does not rise, remove tube and provide artificial ventilation until second attempt can be performed
8. Upon successful placement of tube, auscultate chest to assure proper ventilatory efforts
9. Inflate cuff with 30–35 ml of air and remove syringe
10. Continue to ventilate until:
    a) Other means of ventilation are made (i.e., endotracheal tube), or
    b) Patient begins spontaneous respirations, or
    c) Resuscitation measures are halted

Removal of Tube

1. If patient has been successfully resuscitated or intubated with endotracheal tube (ET), the EOA tube should be removed
2. If condition permits, turn patient onto his side. This step is not necessary if an ET tube is securely in place.
3. Ready suction equipment at bedside. Removal of EOA is always followed by immediate regurgitation.
4. Deflate balloon cuff completely, and carefully withdraw tube

Documentation

Time of insertion, removal of airway, and whether or not endotracheal intubation was performed

Patient's response to resuscitation effort

SUGGESTED READING

American Heart Association. Standards and guidelines for cardiopulmonary resuscitation and emergency cardiac care. JAMA 1986; 255 (21):2934–2935.

American Heart Association. Textbook of advanced cardiac life support. 2nd ed. Dallas: American Heart Association, 1987:29.

Kasen J, Airway management. In: Rosen P, ed. Emergency medicine concepts and clinical practice. Vol. 1. Saint Louis: CV Mosby, 1983:45.

Sheehy SB, Barber J. Basic and advanced life support. In: Sheehy SB, Barber J, eds. Emergency nursing principles and practices. Saint Louis: CV Mosby, 1985:141.

4

ORAL AIRWAY INSERTION

LISA MORRA-MARTIN

Purpose

To maintain an airway in unconscious patients by means of holding the tongue away from the posterior wall of the pharynx

To use as a bite block (when shortened) for patients with endotracheal tubes

Indications

- Seizures prior to the development of tonic or clonic movement
- Unconsciousness
- To maintain an open airway

Contraindications

- Tonic or clonic seizures during which insertion of an airway is nearly impossible without damaging teeth
- Caution should be used when there is extensive oral trauma

Potential Complications

- Damage to mucosa, tongue, or teeth
- Gagging may result in vomiting and lung aspiration if airway is taped in place

Equipment

Oral airway
Tongue depressor (optional depending upon technique used)
1-inch tape

Procedure

1. Wash hands
2. Select oral airway of appropriate size for patient. This may be determined by placing airway on patient's cheek with flat plate at lips. End of airway should be at patient's jaw.
3. Insert airway using one of the following methods:
   a) Invert airway so that tip is facing upward. Begin to slide airway into mouth. As airway approaches the posterior wall of the pharynx near back of the tongue, rotate airway into its proper position (Fig. 4–1).
   b) Using a tongue depressor, move tongue out of the way to avoid pushing tongue backward into posterior pharynx. Insert oral airway into its proper position with tip facing downward. There is no need for rotation.
4. If patient's gag reflex is stimulated, shorten airway slightly and reinsert
5. For use as a bite block, airway may be trimmed so that approximately 2 inches extend beyond the flat plate (in an adult patient)
6. Secure airway with strips of tape placed on cheek and across flat plate of airway, which is at patient's lip. Do not cover opening in airway. Caution should be used to assure that the patient does not gag on the airway when it is taped in place. Taping may prevent patient from being able to dislodge the airway and, therefore, cause the patient to vomit as he regains consciousness.

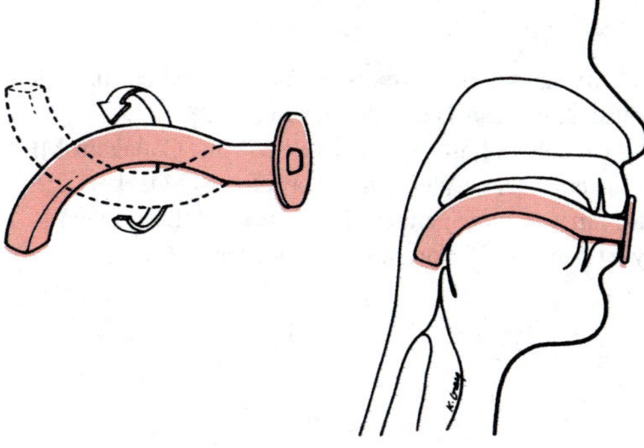

Figure 4–1 Oral airway insertion.

Follow-Up

1. Assess patient's neurologic status frequently. The airway can cause retching and vomiting in a patient who is responsive and should, therefore, be used only in the unconscious patient.
2. Monitor patient for excessive oral secretion and suction oral cavity as necessary
3. If patient's condition permits, long-term maintenance requires removal of the airway to perform mouth care

Documentation

Size of airway used
Time of procedure and patient's tolerance
Any change in patient status and/or any complications
Respiratory rate and character of respiration

SUGGESTED READING

American Heart Association. Textbook of advanced cardiac life support. 2nd ed. Dallas: American Heart Association, 1987:27.

Danzl DF. Principles of airway management. In: Callaham ML, ed. Current therapy in emergency medicine. Toronto: BC Decker, 1987:1.

Stewart RD. Airway management. In: Trunkey DD, Lewis FR, eds. Current therapy of trauma–2. Toronto: BC Decker, 1987:30.

5

THORACENTESIS

LISA A. JONES

Purpose

To remove pleural fluid and/or possibly air by means of a needle puncture through the chest wall into the pleural space. A needle thoracentesis may also be done to detect the presence of blood in the pleural space following chest trauma.

Indications

- Hemothorax
- Pneumothorax
- Pleural effusion
- Empyema
- Hydrothorax

Contraindications

- None

Potential Complications

- Lung damage or reaccumulation of fluid. (Symptoms may include blood-tinged sputum, persistent cough, respiratory distress, or subcutaneous emphysema.)
- Mediastinal shift, if large amounts of fluid are removed. (Symptoms may include those of pulmonary edema or cardiac dis-

tress caused by a sudden shift in mediastinal contents to the side on which the thoracentesis was performed.)
- Infection caused by contamination

Equipment

Small syringe and needle for local anesthesia
Local anesthetic drug
Syringe (50 ml)
Large bore aspirating needle
Three-way stopcock
Sterile tubing
Sterile specimen container
Sterile drapes
Materials for skin preparation
Small sterile dressing
Sterile gloves

Procedure

1. Inform patient about procedure and indicate to patient importance of remaining immobile
2. Position patient sitting upright with neck and dorsal spine flexed and arms and shoulders raised. This may be done by having patient sit on edge of bed and lean over a bedside table with arms folded under his head. If patient is unable to sit, place him on the unaffected side with his arm over his head.
3. Expose entire chest and perform aseptic skin preparation
4. Physician injects local anesthetic into intercostal space with a small gauge needle and syringe. (If fluid is present, the thoracentesis site is usually in the seventh or eighth intercostal space at the posterior axillary line. If air is in the pleural cavity, the site is usually in the second or third intercostal space at the midclavicular line.)

5. The physician then advances the thoracentesis needle, attached to a 50-ml syringe and a three-way stopcock, maintaining constant suction on the syringe, so it is apparent when the fluid pocket is reached
6. Attach sterile tubing to the other end of stopcock and connect tubing to a receptacle
7. When fluid is obtained, turn stopcock adapter open to receptacle for collection of fluid being aspirated. Not more than 1,200 ml should be removed at one time in order to reduce dangers of circulatory collapse or acute pulmonary edema.
8. During procedure, observe patient for difficulty in breathing, tightness in chest, tachypnea, tachycardia, vertigo, hypotension, cyanosis, and diaphoresis
9. After needle is withdrawn, apply pressure over puncture site and then apply a small sterile dressing
10. A needle thoracentesis may also be performed with just needle and syringe in order to detect presence of blood following trauma to chest

Follow-Up

1. Place patient on unaffected side for 1 hour
2. Observe patient for tightness in chest, signs of shock (e.g, faintness, falling blood pressure, and weak rapid pulse), and indications of leakage at puncture site. Also observe patient for signs of lung damage or possible reaccumulation of fluid (blood-tinged sputum, cough, respiratory distress, and subcutaneous emphysema). Watch for indications of mediastinal shift towards the affected side and of pyogenic infection.
3. Frequently, serum electrolyte blood studies are ordered
4. A chest x-ray film may also be ordered to determine effects of procedure

Documentation

Respiratory status and vital signs prior to procedure
Patient and family teaching
Type of skin preparation
Times procedure initiated and completed
Type of anesthetic used and any allergies
Total amount, color, and character of fluid removed
Any complications during procedure
Respiratory status (breath sounds) and vital signs following
  procedures
Any complications following procedures
Sterile dressing applied to site

SUGGESTED READING

Brunner L, Suddarth D. The Lippincott manual of nursing practice. Philadelphia: JB Lippincott, 1974:122.
Tucker S. Patient care standards. Saint Louis: CV Mosby, 1975:76.
Luckman J, Sorenson K. Diagnosis and evaluation of the patient with a respiratory disorder. In: Luckman J, Sorenson K, eds. Medical-surgical nursing. 1st ed. Philadelphia: WB Saunders, 1974:865.

6

TRACHEOSTOMY

BARBARA CLARK MIMS

Purpose

To establish a patent airway

Indications

- Upper airway obstruction
- Prolonged mechanical ventilation
- Need for intensive pulmonary hygiene

Contraindications

- None

Potential Complications

- Infection
- Ulceration of tracheal mucosa
- Tracheal dilatation
- Tracheal stenosis
- Tracheal malacia
- Tracheoesophageal fistula
- Hemorrhage
- Pneumothorax
- Damage to laryngeal nerve
- Airway obstruction (crusting of secretions, herniation of cuff, kinking of tube)

Equipment

Tracheostomy tray:
- 2% lidocaine (with or without epinephrine, depending on physician's preference)
- Sterile towels
- Surgical attire (sterile gowns, gloves, caps, and masks)
- Syringes (10ml) (2)
- #25 gauge needle
- Sheet roll
- Suture (usually 2–0 chromic and 2–0 silk)

Iodophor solution
10-pack 4 × 4 gauze sponges
Tracheostomy tubes (2 of size physician orders, 1 of size smaller, 1 of size larger)
Suction apparatus
Sterile suction catheter and glove
Sterile Yankauer suction tip
Sterile sheet
Oxygen setup or ventilator as ordered

Procedure

1. If patient is conscious, physician should explain procedure and obtain operative permit
2. Assure that patient has a patent intravenous (IV). (There may be a need to administer narcotics for sedation or emergency drugs during procedure.)
3. Assemble crash cart and other equipment at bedside. Ask physician what type of suture is preferred and what size tube is to be used.
4. Check to be sure suction equipment and ambu bag are set up and functioning
5. If patient is not on a cardiac monitor, connect either to a monitor or to an electrocardiograph machine

6. Remove head of bed or stretcher
7. Assist physician(s) in donning sterile gown(s), glove(s), cap(s), and mask(s)
8. Position sheet roll between patient's shoulder blades
9. Open sterile towels and sheet and hand to physician, who then drapes patient
10. Open 10-pack of 4 × 4 sponges and pass to physician
11. Open package and pass 10-ml syringe to physician in sterile manner
12. Connect #25 gauge needle to syringe that is in physician's hand. Maintain sterile technique.
13. Cleanse tip of 2% lidocaine bottle with iodophor preparation
14. Invert bottle of 2% lidocaine so that physician may insert needle and aspirate 10 ml into syringe
15. Open tracheostomy tray. Position tray on overbed table within physician's reach.
16. Open suture material and tracheostomy tube and place on tracheostomy tray
17. Make certain that physician checks the cuff for symmetrical expansion and leaks
18. If patient is intubated with an endotracheal tube (ET), the physician may ask the nurse to slowly withdraw ET tube as he inserts tracheostomy tube. Be sure to suction nasopharynx and mouth and deflate cuff before withdrawing tube.
19. Support and comfort patient throughout procedure. Keep IV line accessible in case drugs need to be administered and watch monitor for dysrhythmias.
20. Once tube is in place, physician may or may not suture it to skin. The nurse secures it in place with tracheostomy tape.
21. Once tube is in place, inflate cuff with the minimal occlusive volume (see *Endotracheal Intubation*), ventilate patient, and auscultate breath sounds to assess adequacy of ventilation
22. Suction tube

Follow-Up

1. Apply oxygen and set up a ventilator as ordered
2. Apply a sterile dressing around insertion site. Do not use cotton-filled flats and do not cut 4 × 4 gauze sponge. These may result in bits of fiber being aspirated.
3. Order a stat portable chest x-ray film to verify tube placement and to check for pneumothorax
4. Clean patient and provide comfort measures as indicated
5. Tape identical size and type of tracheostomy tube to head of bed

Documentation

Name(s) of physician(s) that performed procedure
Size and type of tracheostomy tube
Amount of air needed to establish minimal occlusive volume
Patient's tolerance of procedure
Route and percentage of oxygen administered or ventilator settings

SUGGESTED READING

Abels LF. Mosby's manual of critical care. Saint Louis: CV Mosby 1979:142.
Morrison ML. Respiratory intensive care nursing. 2nd ed. Boston: Little, Brown, 1980:99.
Persons CB. Critical care procedures and protocols. A nursing process approach. Philadelphia: JB Lippincott, 1987:255.
Smith S, Duell D. Clinical nursing skills. Los Altos: National Nursing Review, 1985:674.

7

TUBE THORACOSTOMY

JORIE SCOTT

Purpose

To reestablish negative pressure in chest
To reinflate lung
To evacuate fluid accumulation in chest

Indications

- Pneumothorax
- Hemothorax
- Prophylaxis, in selected cases of suspected severe lung injury
- Pulmonary restriction

Diagnostic and therapeutic approach to chest trauma is the same for children as adults. However, a child's wall is extremely compliant and allows energy to transfer to the interthoracic structures, frequently without any evidence of injury on the internal chest wall. Tension pneumothorax or hemopneumothorax are not well tolerated by the child because of mobility of the mediastinal structures. This also makes the child especially sensitive to flail segments.

Contraindications

- None

Potential Complications

- Intercostal bleeding
- Empyema (1-16% of cases develop empyema)
- Damage to intercostal nerve, vein, or artery
- Damage to mammary vessels
- Mediastinal emphysema
- Reoccurrence of pneumothorax

Equipment

Betadine
4 × 4 gauze sponges
Light sources
Sedation if indicated
Lidocaine 1% without epinephrine (20ml)
Syringe (10ml), #18 and #23 gauge needle
Chest tube—28 or 36 French (for adult)
Chest drainage system, suction (Emerson pump)
Supplemental oxygen
Thoracostomy tray:
    Sterile drapes
    Scalpel blade and handle—#10 and #11
    Needle holders (4)
Small tinochette chest retractor or small self retaining chest retractor (2)
Mosquito clamps (6)
Large curved Kelly clamps (4)
Heavy curved scissors (2)
Suture scissors (2)
Metsenbaum curved dissecting scissors (2)
Tissue forceps with and without teeth (2)
Benzoin solution

Tape
Suture:
    2-0, 30 silk cutting needle
    2-0, 30 silk with taper needle
    4-0 monofilament with noncutting needle

Procedure

1. Assess patient's airway, breathing, and circulation (ABCs)
2. Intervene to protect ABCs
3. Administer supplemental oxygen as needed
4. Establish intravenous access and ensure adequate fluid resuscitation
5. Assess patient and suspect underlying chest injury if any of the following are noted:
    a) Bruising across chest or abdomen
    b) Entrance or exit wound mark
    c) Asymmetry of the chest
    d) Use of accessory muscle for respiration
    e) Retractions
    f) Absence of breath sounds, hyperresonance
    g) Sternum anterolateral ribcage fractures
    h) Pain
    i) Presence of subcutaneous emphysema
6. Notify physician if patient develops respiratory complications
7. Obtain baseline arterial blood gases (ABGs)
8. Notify respiratory therapist if needed
9. If possible, determine if patient is allergic to betadine
10. If time allows, explain procedure to patient and family
11. Place on cardiac monitor
12. Position patient by placing in a supine position with a sheet roll under affected side at shoulder level. Place arm over head and restrain patient if indicated.

13. Sedate patient if indicated. Caution must be exhibited because of possible respiratory depression.
14. Assist physician with preparation of the area. Have betadine and 4 × 4 sponges available.
15. Direct light source to appropriate chest side
16. Assist physician in anesthetizing area
17. Assist physician in gloving, masking, and gowning
18. Open chest tube tray
19. Assist physician in establishing sterile field
20. Open chest tube of indicated size onto sterile field
21. Open suture material
22. Open and assemble chest drainage system
23. Set suction apparatus initially to 20 cm of suction
24. Assist physician in inserting tube (Fig. 7-1)
25. Assess for proper tube placement by noting fogging of chest tube with expiration and by listening for air movement
26. Note amount and consistency of initial chest tube output

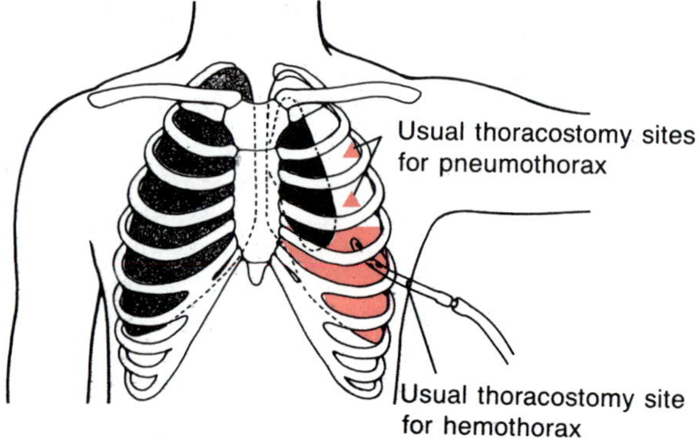

Figure 7-1 Tube placements for a thoracostomy.

27. Connect chest tube to chest drainage system, and note immediate output
28. Connect chest drainage system to suction at 20 cm of water suction
29. Alert Operating Room if further surgical intervention is indicated. (Note: a 1,500 ml initial loss or a 1,000 ml loss followed by a loss of 200 ml/hr for 4 hours indicates a massive hemothorax that needs surgical intervention.)
30. Assist physician in suturing chest tube in place
31. Assist physician in applying dressing
32. Call for immediate x-ray film to check chest tube placement
33. Assist physician in readjusting tube placement if indicated

Follow-Up

1. Assess respiratory adequacy by observing for changes in respiratory rate or rhythm, symmetry of chest, use of accessory or intercostal muscles, or retraction
2. Auscultate for bilateral breath sounds and hyperresonance
3. Observe for onset of an increase in the presence of subcutaneous emphysema. This may indicate an air leak in the system which needs further evaluation.
4. Note any changes in level of consciousness or skin color
5. Monitor vital signs and chest drainage output q15min ×4, q30min ×2, then q1h until stable
6. Monitor chest drainage q1h
7. Continue with head-to-toe examination and evaluation
8. Intervene as indicated

Documentation

Initial assessment of patient
Procedure and outcome
Ongoing respiratory assessment

SUGGESTED READING

American College of Surgeons Committee on Trauma. Advanced trauma life support. Chicago: American College of Surgeons, 1985:73.

Graham JM, Matlox KL, Deal AC Jr. Penetrating trauma of the lung. J Trauma 1979;19:665.

Simoneau JK. Nursing process in cardiac trauma emergencies. In: Holloway NM, ed. Emergency department nurses association. Core curriculum. Philadelphia: WB Saunders, 1985:161.

CARDIAC PROCEDURES

8

CARDIAC MONITORING

LAURA LUECKE

Purpose

To provide data regarding electrical cardiac activity

Indications

- To provide early detection of cardiac dysrhythmias

Contraindications

- None

Potential Complications

- Altered skin integrity. (If irritation observed, clean site and re-apply electrode at new site. If patient is allergic to electrode adhesive, apply nonallergic electrodes.)
- Electromicroshock. (Follow electrical safety guidelines. Avoid using equipment without current inspection sticker. Be sure that equipment is properly grounded. Do not use equipment with frayed cords, broken connectors, or broken plugs.)
- Equipment malfunction

Equipment

Electrocardiogram (ECG) monitoring system
Electrodes (pregelled disposable electrodes or nondisposable electrodes and electrode gel)
Razor
Alcohol preparation pads
Gauze pads

Procedure

1. Explain procedure to patient and answer all questions
2. Prepare ECG monitoring system as directed by manufacturer
3. Turn ECG monitor on (some units require a short warm-up period). Turn alarms off.
4. Choose sites for electrode placement (two common sites are shown in Figure 8–1):
   a) Lead II – This lead is utilized for a positive tall QRS and P wave. It cannot be utilized to distinguish between right and left bundle branch block patterns.
      (1) Apply negative electrode to first intercostal space, right sternal border
      (2) Apply positive electrode to fourth intercostal space, left midclavicular line
      (3) If a three-lead system is used, apply ground electrode just below left clavicle, midclavicular line
   b) MCL_1 (modified chest lead V_1) – This lead produces a negative QRS complex and a P wave of variable polarity. It is best utilized for identification of bundle branch blocks and for differential diagnosis of ventricular ectopy. Electrode placement does not interfere with auscultation or defibrillation.
      (1) Apply negative electrode just below left clavicle, midclavicular line

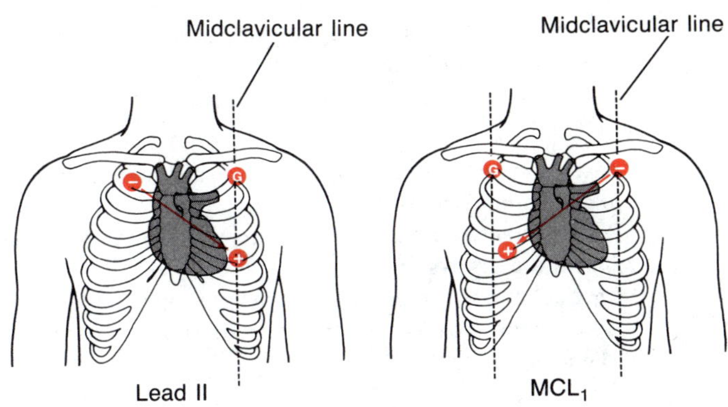

Figure 8–1 Sites for electrode placement for cardiac monitoring.

> (2) Apply positive electrode at fourth intercostal space, right sternal border
>
> (3) If a three-lead system is used, apply ground electrode just below right clavicle, midclavicular line

5. Shave area if needed to minimize discomfort or facilitate conduction

6. Clean sites with an alcohol preparation pad. Rub sites dry with gauze pads and abrade skin slightly.

7. Connect electrodes to lead wires

8. Peel paper backing off electrode and check to be sure conduction jelly is present

9. Place patches on intended sites, applying pressure in a circular pattern around edges of electrode. Do not press on center of electrode, as this may cause displacement of gel and poor adhesive contact.

10. Examine ECG. The R wave should be twice the height of the other wave form components.

11. Turn alarms on, and set rate according to hospital policy

12. Test alarm system according to manufacturer's instructions
13. Obtain a rhythm strip

Follow-Up

1. Assess rhythm strip for dysrhythmias, and provide prompt intervention as necessary
2. Perform continuous ECG monitor surveillance, and check that alarms are always on
3. Check electrode contact, and be sure that there is sufficient gel
4. Assess skin integrity. Rotate electrode sites as needed.
5. Maintain a clear ECG recording

Trouble Shooting

- Wandering ECG baseline (Fig. 8–2a)
  - Possible causes:
    a) Patient movement
    b) Poor electrode contact
    c) Tension on electrode and lead wires
    d) Movement of cable with respirations
  - Possible interventions:
    a) Assess patient for discomfort or anxiety
    b) Check electrodes and lead wires
    c) Move cable off chest wall. May move left lower patch to a more lateral position to minimize respiratory movement interference.

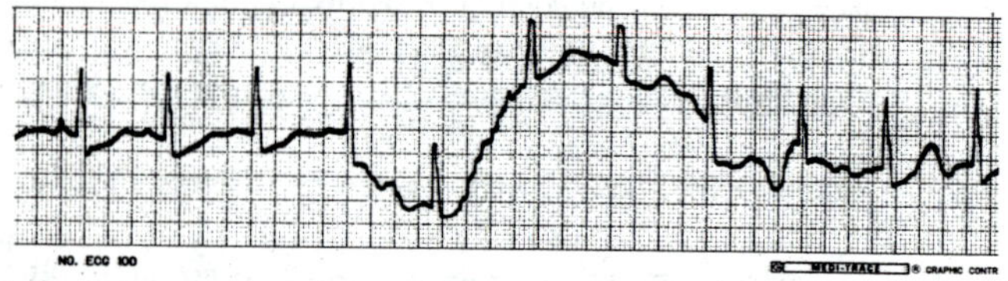

Figure 8–2a Wandering ECG baseline.

- Electrical (60-cycle) interference (Fig. 8–2b)
  - □ Possible causes:
    - a) Electrical interference from other equipment in the room
    - b) Improper electrical equipment grounding
    - c) X-ray or diathermy equipment in operation
  - □ Possible interventions:
    - a) Assure that equipment is grounded
    - b) Isolate source by systematically unplugging and reconnecting electrical machines around bedside (one at a time) until interference ceases

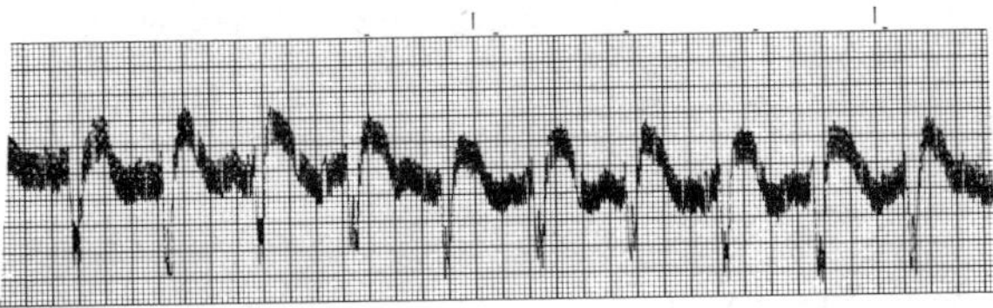

Figure 8–2b Electrical interference (60-cycle artifact).

- Artifact (Fig. 8–2c)
  - □ Possible causes:
    - a) Poor electrode contact
    - b) Patient movement
  - □ Possible interventions:
    - a) Check electrodes and lead wires
    - b) Assess patient for discomfort or anxiety
    - c) Reposition electrodes and/or lead wires to areas with less muscle movement

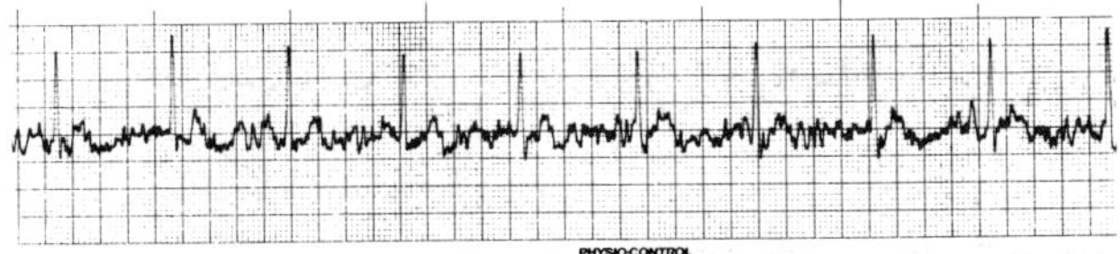

Figure 8–2c Excessive artifact.

- False low rate alarm triggering (Fig. 8–2d)
  - □ Possible causes:
    - a) QRS complex too small to register
    - b) Low rate alarm set too low
    - c) Wandering baseline or artifact
  - □ Possible interventions:
    - a) Assess patient movement
    - b) Check electrodes and lead wires
    - c) Adjust leads or monitor controls to obtain a taller R wave
    - d) Set alarm limits according to patient's heart rate

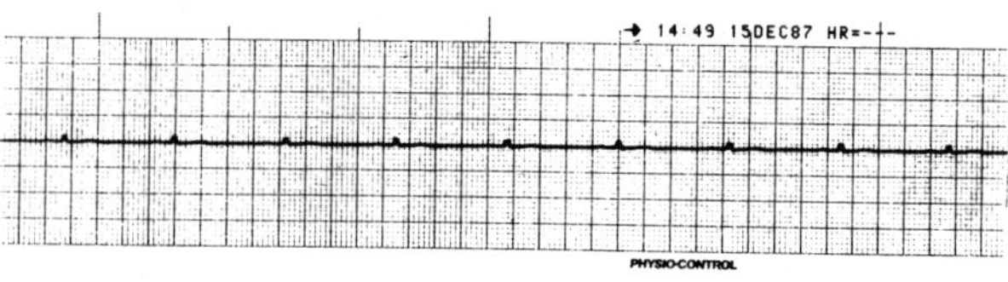

Figure 8–2d False low alarm.

- False high alarm triggering (Fig. 8–2e)
  - □ Possible causes:
    - a) Double triggering. P wave or T wave and QRS are of equal height, causing monitor to sense both waves and falsely to double the rate.
    - b) Artifact sensed by monitor as a QRS complex, falsely evaluating the rate
    - c) High rate alarm set too high

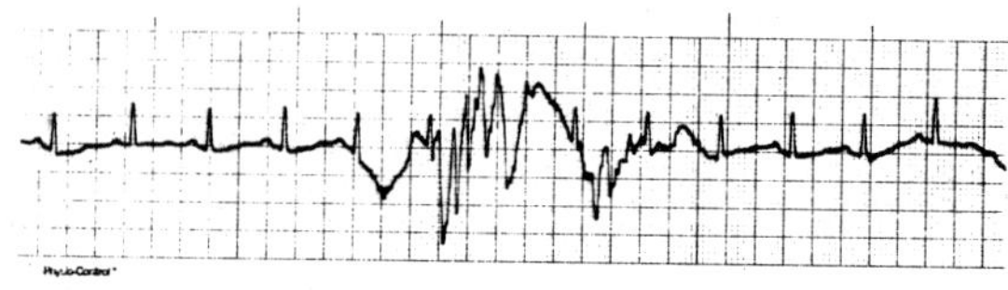

Figure 8–2e False high alarm.

- Possible interventions:
  - a) Assess patient movement
  - b) Check electrodes and leadwires
  - c) Adjust leads or monitor controls so that R wave is twice the height of P wave and T wave
  - d) Set alarm limits according to patient's heart rate

Documentation

Initial rhythm and lead used
That alarms are on and functioning
Other observations of patient's condition
Any dysrhythmias observed and interventions performed

SUGGESTED READING

Andreoli KG, Fowkes VH, Zipes DP, Wallace AG. Comprehensive cardiac care. 4th ed. Saint Louis: CV Mosby, 1979:463.

Elsden A, Mutton A. Nursing photobook series - using monitors. In: West R, ed. Nursing 80. Horsham, PA: Intermed Communications, 1981:50.

Millar S, Sampson LK, Soukup M. AACN Procedure manual for critical care. Philadelphia: WB Saunders, 1985:16.

9

TRANSCUTANEOUS CARDIAC PACING

MOLLY A. SEAMAN

Purpose

To provide electrical stimulation to the myocardium to regain normal cardiac function

Indications

- Symptomatic bradycardia
- Need for overdrive pacing for atrial or ventricular tachyarrhythmias
- Need for prophylactic pacing in acute myocardial infarction

Contraindications

- The literature is not in agreement on contraindications

Potential Complications

- Erythema
- Dysrhythmia
- Pain
- Tissue damage

Equipment

Pacing device
8–cm conducting electrodes (2)

Procedure

1. Maintain patient's airway, breathing, and circulation. Have emergency cart at bedside.
2. If patient awake, explain procedure and what to expect. Physician may also consider mild sedation during procedure if indicated.
3. Dry patient's skin on anterior and posterior skin surface
4. Apply posterior electrode at level of heart between scapula and spine
5. The anterior electrode is placed as close as possible to the point of maximal impulse (PMI) between fourth and fifth ribs
6. Connect patient to cardiac monitor (leaving space in case defibrillation is needed)
7. Attach pacing electrodes to output cable of pacing device
8. The rate and pulse duration are fixed on the unit, but physician determines milliampere (MA) (output) settings
9. The unit should be on and in *pace* mode
10. Observe monitor for capture. Assess presence or absence of peripheral pulses with pacing.

Follow-Up

1. Continue to monitor patient's cardiovascular status
2. Prepare patient for further definitive treatment

Documentation

Patient's status before, during, and after pacing
Type of pacing unit and output (in MAs) required for capture
Time of placement
Disposition of patient, whether admitted to cardiac unit or fluoroscopy for further treatment

SUGGESTED READING

Cooper PR. A guide to external pacing. RN 1987; 3:48–49.

Roberts JR, Syverud SA. Emergency pacemaker insertion and malfunction. In: Callaham ML, ed. Current therapy in emergency medicine. Toronto: BC Decker, 1987:465.

Roberts JR. Transthoracic, transcutaneous cardiac pacing. In: Roberts JR, Hedges JR, eds. Clinical procedures in emergency medicine. Philadelphia: WB Saunders 1985:201.

10

TRANSTHORACIC CARDIAC PACING

MOLLY A. SEAMAN

Purpose

To provide electrical stimulation to the myocardium to regain normal cardiac function

Indications

- Asystole
- Profound bradycardias
- Heart blocks (unstable or high degree)
- Recurrent ventricular tachycardias

Contraindications

- Patients who are stable and/or awake
- Any cardiac condition that is easily managed by drug therapy
- Electromechanical dissociation
- Ventricular fibrillation

Potential Complications

- Pneumothorax
- Pericardial tamponade
- Emboli
- Sepsis
- Laceration to myocardium or coronary artery

Equipment

Pulse generator
Transthoracic pacing kit
If self contained kit not available, use the following:
    Povidone-iodine solution
    30–37-cm bipolar pacing wire
    13-cm, #18 gauge steel needle (introducer)
    Syringe (10 ml)
    Plastic electrical connector
    Sterile gloves

Procedure

1. Maintain patient's airway, breathing, circulation until insertion of pacer is possible
2. Connect patient to cardiac monitor
3. Make sure that patient has a patent intravenous (IV) line
4. Test pulse generator to ensure it is sensing. Replace battery if needed.
5. Have emergency equipment and drugs ready
6. Assist physician with catheter insertion
7. Monitor patient's rhythm and vital signs continuously
8. Once pacing wire is positioned, attach end of wire to plastic electrical connector
9. Securely attach negative and positive leads from plastic electrical connector to appropriate terminals on pulse generator
10. With the pulse generator in the fixed or asynchronous mode, observe monitor for a pacer spike
11. The settings should be made according to physician's orders. In general, the rate should be set between 70–90 beats per minute. The ouput control should be turned to the maximum milliampere (MA) that provides capture.
12. Apply sterile dressing to site and secure pulse generator next to patient

Follow-Up

1. Once patient is stable obtain chest x-ray film and 12-lead electrocardiogram
2. Prepare for insertion of transvenous or permanent pacemaker

Documentation

All settings: mode, output (in MAs) rate, and type of pacing wire
Patient's response to pacer wire insertion
Patient's condition before and after insertion. Document these findings, noting level of consciousness, vital signs, skin color, and skin temperature.

SUGGESTING READING

American Heart Association. Textbook of advance cardiac life support. 2nd ed. Dallas: American Heart Association, 1987:192.

Braun AE. Transthoracic pacing in the emergency department. J Emerg Nurs 1986; 12:354–359.

Roberts JR. Transthoracic, transcutaneous cardiac pacing. In: Roberts JR, Hedges JR, eds. Clinical procedure in emergency medicine. Philadelphia: WB Saunders, 1985:191.

11

TRANSVENOUS CARDIAC PACING

MOLLY A. SEAMAN

Purpose

To provide electrical stimulation to the myocardium to regain normal cardiac function

Indications

- Bradycardias
  - □ Sick sinus syndrome
  - □ 2nd and 3rd degree heart block
  - □ Atrial fibrillation with slow ventricular response
  - □ Left and/or right bundle branch block, bifascicular block, hemiblocks in the face of myocardial infarction
- Tachycardias
  - □ Supraventricular
  - □ Ventricular
  - □ Atrial flutter

Contraindications

- Unclear of benefits in asystolic arrest

Potential Complications

- Arrhythmias
- Cardiac perforation
- Emboli
- Infection
- Pneumothorax

Equipment

Pulse generator and connecting cable
#5 French balloon tipped bipolar pacing catheter with syringe
Electrocardiogram machine
Percutaneous catheter sheath introducer
Sterile gloves, masks
Povidone-iodine solution

Procedure

1. Test pulse generator prior to insertion
2. Gather insertion equipment at bedside
3. Have emergency cart and drugs available
4. Assure airway, breathing, and circulation
5. Establish intravenous (IV) line at keep open rate
6. If patient awake, explain procedure
7. Prepare area of insertion as indicated. Most common transvenous access sites are the brachial and femoral approaches.
8. Assist physician during line insertion
9. Monitor patients rhythm continuously
10. Once pacing catheter is introduced 10–12 cm, connect the distal end to the pulse generator, making sure all connections are secure and in appropriate terminals
11. Turn unit on to sense, but not to pace
12. The physician gives order for setting rate and output controls on pulse generator

13. The pulse generator should be placed in the synchronous mode. Rate is usually 80–90 beats per minute. During emergency blind insertion the milliampere (MA) is turned to the maximum amperes until capture is obtained.
14. Controls can be adjusted according to patient's response
15. A secured sterile dressing should be placed on insertion site after catheter properly positioned. Secure pulse generator to patient's arm.
16. Prepare to admit patient to intensive care

Follow-Up

1. Continue to monitor all vitals signs and level of consciousness
2. Monitor rhythm closely and be prepared to treat dysrhythmias
3. Offer reassurance to awake patient
4. Make sure all equipment is electrically safe and be aware of possible microshocks

Documentation

All rhythms before, during, and after insertion
Patient's cardiovascular status before, during, and after insertion
All settings used to first gain capture; recording mode, rate, and MAs
Any emergency drugs used

SUGGESTED READING

American Heart Association. Textbook of advanced cardiac life support. 2nd ed. Dallas: American Heart Association, 1987:187.
Benjamin GC. Emergency transvenous cardiac pacing. In: Roberts JR, Hedges

JR, eds. Clinical procedures in emergency medicine. Philadelphia: WB Saunders 1985:164.

Roberts JR, Syverud SA. Emergency pacemaker insertion and malfunction. In: Callaham ML, ed. Current therapy in emergency medicine. Toronto: BC Decker, 1987:465.

12

CARDIOVERSION

KATHLEEN H. TOTO

Purpose

To convert ventricular and supraventricular tachydysrhythmias to sinus rhythm by means of synchronized electrical depolarization of the myocardium

Indications

- Elective cardioversion is indicated for treatment of stable supraventricular tachydysrhythmias that are unresponsive to medical therapy. Example: paroxysmal atrial tachycardia (PAT), atrial fibrillation, atrial flutter, junctional tachycardia.
- Emergency cardioversion is indicated for treatment of ventricular and supraventricular tachydysrhythmias that are unstable and must be terminated immediately to prevent hemodynamic deterioration

Contraindications

- Digitalis toxicity. (Cardioversion and defibrillation enhance effects of digitalis and may result in lethal dysrhythmias. Patients on maintenance doses of digitalis usually should have their digitalis held for at least 24 hours prior to elective cardioversion. Emergency cardioversion is usually not indicated for digitalis toxic dysrhythmias.)

- Hypokalemia. (Serum potassium levels should be evaluated prior to elective cardioversion as hypokalemia enhances electrical instability and may precipitate postconversion dysrhythmias.)

Potential Complications

- Ventricular fibrillation. (If the patient goes into ventricular fibrillation, turn synchronizing mode OFF and defibrillate immediately with 200 watt seconds)
- Respiratory depression or arrest from oversedation
- Pulmonary or systemic emboli
- Skin burns

Equipment

Cardioverter-defibrillator
Electrocardiogram (ECG) monitor
12-lead ECG machine
Conductive medium (ECG gel or paste or normal saline soaked
   4 × 4 sponges)
Cardiac arrest cart
Suction equipment
Ambu bag
Oxygen therapy
Airway
Emergency pacing equipment

Procedure

1. Assure that signed permit is on chart for elective cardioversion and that patient is aware of what to expect
2. Evaluate patient's recent serum electrolyte levels and digitalis level, if appropriate

3. Evaluate patient's medication record to be sure patient has not received digitalis within the last 24 hours. If the patient has received digitalis within the last 24 hours, this would not necessarily preclude cardioversion. However, the physician should be notified.

4. Assure patient has had nothing by mouth for approximately 8 hours prior to elective cardioversion

5. Obtain a baseline 12-lead ECG of patient's rhythm

6. Assess patient's intravenous (IV) line to assure patency. (If an IV is not in place, insert one before proceeding.)

7. Place patient in supine position to assure proper placement of paddles

8. Assess patient's vital signs, level of orientation, respiratory status, and peripheral pulses

9. Remove dentures or dental prosthesis. (This reduces the risk of airway obstruction, but is not always appropriate as dentures may also enhance airway support.)

10. Administer oxygen therapy as ordered prior to cardioversion, and discontinue oxygen at the time of cardioversion as it is potentially combustible with electrical arching

11. Prepare equipment for cardioversion:
    a) Plug defibrillator into electrical outlet, even if battery operated
    b) Turn power on
    c) Connect patient to limb leads of monitor-cardioverter. Assure that monitoring lead produces a tall, upright R wave (in some newer models it is not necessary for R wave to be upright to be sensed by cardioverter). Assure R wave is of sufficient amplitude to trigger synchronizing circuit of cardioverter.
    d) Check monitor for artifact. (If artifact is present, check electrode placement and/or contact and alter as needed to assure no artifact is present. Artifact may be interpret-

ed by the cardioverter as an R wave and could allow electrical current to be delivered at incorrect time, which could result in ventricular fibrillation.)

   e) Activate synchronizer. (If synchronizer is not activated, electrical discharge will occur when paddle buttons are depressed regardless of R wave.)

   f) Check synchronizing circuit. (Most units have a light that flashes on the R wave or may have an auditory tone that beeps with the R wave to demonstrate the cardioverter is *in synchrony* with patient's cardiac cycle.)

12. Administer sedation as prescribed. Intravenous Valium in gradated doses of 5 – 10 mg may be given because cardioversion is painful and anxiety-producing. A short-acting anesthetic may also be given. (When this is done, an anesthesiologist should be in attendance to monitor airway and respirations.)

13. Cover entire paddle surface with conductive medium

14. Select energy level on cardioverter. The joules will be prescribed by the physician based on the patient's body weight, dysrhythmia, and medications. The American Heart Association recommends the following:

    a) Atrial fibrillation: 100 joules

    b) Atrial flutter: 25 joules

    c) Paroxysmal supraventricular tachycardia (PSVT): 75–100 joules

    d) Unstable ventricular tachycardia (with a pulse): 50 joules

15. Activate charge button on machine or on paddles

16. Assure cardioverter is fully charged to the set level

17. Assure patient's chest is free of any moisture because this may cause arching and decreased energy delivery to the myocardium

18. Place paddles firmly on patient's chest using 25 pounds of pressure per paddle:
    a) Standard placement. Place one paddle to right of sternum below clavicle. Place other paddle to left of left nipple in anterior axillary line.
    b) Anterior-posterior placement. Place one paddle at posterior intrascapular area. Place other paddle at anterior precordial area.
19. Check rhythm on ECG monitor, and double check that synchronizer has been activated and is firing on the R wave
20. Stand clear of bed, and command others to stand clear of bed
21. Depress discharge buttons
22. Check patient's pulse and vital signs. Assess postcardioversion ECG rhythm.
23. Repeat steps 13 through 22 as needed to terminate tachydysrhythmia. (If rhythm persists, the energy level should be increased in increments as prescribed by physician. When repeated shocks are given, the interval between shocks should be at least 3 minutes. Ensure that adequate conductive medium is on paddles for repeated countershocks.)
24. Check equipment for potential causes of failure to cardiovert:
    a) Nonsynchronized mode
    b) Artifact interference
    c) Battery failure (if not plugged in)
    d) Inadequate pressure on paddles during cardioversion

Follow-Up

1. Postcardioversion assessment:
   a) ECG rhythm
   b) Vital signs
   c) Airway patency
   d) Respirations

2. Orient patient to surroundings and results of cardioversion
3. Assess patient for chest burns, and treat as necessary
4. Obtain a postcardioversion 12-lead ECG to assess for myocardial damage
5. Monitor patient's ECG continuously for at least 2 hours post-procedure

Documentation

Patient's status prior to cardioversion:
    Vital signs
    Level of consciousness
    Pulses
    Respirations (rate and depth)
    ECG rhythm
    Presence of patent IV line
    Name, dose, and route of sedation administered
Sequence of cardioversions:
    ECG rhythm prior to each shock
    Time and amount of energy delivered with each shock
    Postcardioversion ECG rhythm
Patient's status following procedure:
    Vital signs
    Level of consciousness
    Pulses
    Respirations (rate and depth)
    ECG rhythm

SUGGESTED READINGS

American Heart Association. Textbook of advanced cardiac life support. 2nd ed. Dallas: American Heart Association, 1987:92,244.

Hudak CM, Gallo BM, Lohr T. Critical care nursing. 4th ed. Philadelphia: JB Lippincott, 1986:167.

Kenner CV, Guzetta CE, Dossey BM. Critical care nursing: body, mind, spirit. 2nd ed. Boston: Little, Brown, 1985:452.

Millar S, Sampson LK, Soukup M, eds. AACN Procedure manual for critical care. 1st ed. Philadelphia: WB Saunders 1985:29.

13

DEFIBRILLATION

MARY E. MANCINI

Purpose

To terminate ventricular fibrillation by means of an electrical discharge across the patient's chest wall. Early defibrillation has been shown to significantly increase the likelihood of successful resuscitation.

Indications

- Ventricular fibrillation
- Ventricular tachycardia when the patient is unconscious and pulseless
- If there is a possibility that what appears to be asystole may actually be fine ventricular fibrillation

Contraindications

- None

Potential Complications

- Skin burn from defibrillator paddles
- Damage to myocardium

Equipment

Defibrillator
Electrode paste
Electrocardiogram (ECG) machine
Cardiac arrest cart
Wall suction or suction machine
Cardiopulmonary resuscitation (CPR) record

Procedure

1. Assess patient to assure patient is pulseless
2. Position defibrillator so that paddles can easily reach patient's chest
3. Plug defibrillator into electrical outlet. (If defibrillator is battery operated and electrical outlet is available, plug in so as to prevent premature emptying of batteries.)
4. Push power button in, and be sure indicator light is on. Most units have a synchronization circuit which must be in the *off* or inoperative mode for treatment of ventricular fibrillation.
5. Cover entire paddle surface with thin coat of electrode paste (or, if available, place prepackaged defibrillation pads on chest)
6. Select correct energy level on machine. Initial defibrillation attempt should be in the range of 200–300 joules delivered energy.
7. Press charge button either on machine or on paddles themselves
8. Watch charge meter needle until it shows the specified charge, listen for alarm that indicates a full charge
9. Wipe all moisture from diaphoresis or solutions off patient's chest
10. Position paddles on chest with firm, even pressure. Place one paddle just to right of upper sternum and below clavicle and

the other just to left of apex of heart and midaxillary line. The V_1 and V_6 electrode positions of the 12-lead ECG have been shown to be effective (Fig. 13–1).

11. The operator directs all personnel to stand clear and release hold on any equipment that is in contact with patient or bed. The operator should look to assure everyone is clear of bed.
12. Apply greater than 20 pounds pressure on paddles, and simultaneously depress knobs on paddles to release electrical charge
13. Check the patient's pulse
14. Assess postdefibrillation ECG pattern. Continue CPR during any delays.
15. If ventricular fibrillation continues, immediately repeat steps 6 through 14. Ensure that adequate electrode paste is on paddles for each defibrillation.
16. If ventricular fibrillation continues, repeat steps 6 through 14 at up to 360 joules
17. If third defibrillation is unsuccessful, resume CPR and initiate appropriate Advanced Cardiac Life Support algorithm

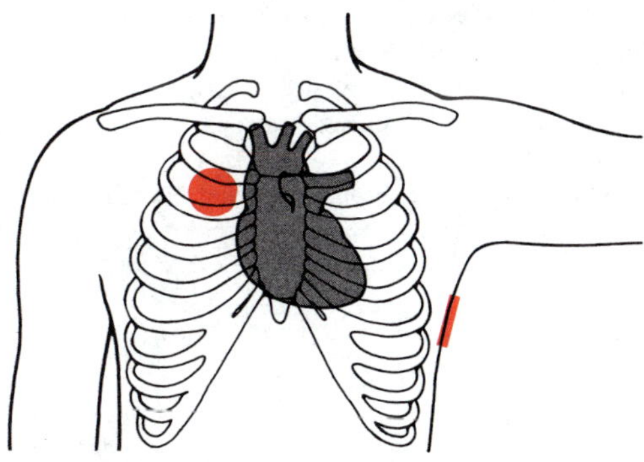

Figure 13–1 Paddle placement for defibrillation.

Follow-Up

1. Assess patient for burns and treat, if necessary
2. Clean lubricant off patient's chest and paddles
3. Monitor, report, and record vital signs frequently until condition is stable

Documentation

Character of cardiac rhythm and patient's clinical condition prior to defibrillation

Time and amount of energy delivered for each defibrillation

Time of physician's arrival

Cardiac rhythm and patient's physical (and psychological, if applicable) condition in response to procedure

SUGGESTED READING

American Heart Association. Standards and guidelines for cardiopulmonary resuscitation and emergency cardiac care. JAMA 1986; 255 (21): 2841–3044.

Brunner LS, Suddarth DS, eds. The Lippincott manual of nursing practice. 3rd ed. Philadelphia: JB Lippincott, 1982:277.

Niemann JT. Improving systemic perfusion during cardiopulmonary resuscitation. In: Callaham ML, ed. Current therapy in emergency medicine. Toronto: BC Decker, 1987:43.

Pepe PE, Hudson LD. Acute respiratory failure. In: Callaham ML, ed. Current therapy in emergency medicine. Toronto: BC Decker, 1987:30.

14

ELECTROCARDIOGRAM: 12 LEAD

KAREN KRENTZ

Purpose

To obtain a record for interpretation and documentation of cardiac electrical activity

Indications

- Identification of damaged areas of the myocardium, dysrhythmias, intraventricular conduction defects, and other abnormalities

Contraindications

- Combative or uncooperative patient

Complications

- None

Equipment

Electrocardiogram (ECG) machine (single or multiple channeled) including four limb electrodes with rubber straps and chest electrodes
Electrode gel

Procedure

1. Prepare ECG recorder by placing it at bedside, plugging it into a grounded outlet, and turning on power

2. Prepare patient by explaining procedure. Assure patient that the procedure is painless and will only take a few minutes. Place patient in a supine position with arms, legs, and chest exposed.

3. Attach limb leads to each extremity distally. Choose a flat, fleshy site to secure electrode straps. Apply electrode gel to each electrode plate, and make sure electrodes are firmly attached.

4. Attach limb lead wires to appropriate limb plate. Each wire is labeled and color coded for easy identification.

5. Identify placement of chest leads and mark with electrode gel or ink (Fig. 14-1):

   (Chest Lead) V_1 - 4th intercostal space, right sternal border

                           V_2 - 4th intercostal space, left sternal border

                           V_3 - 5th intercostal space, midway between V_2 and V_4

                           V_4 - 5th intercostal space, midclavicular line

                           V_5 - 5th intercostal space, left anterior axillary line

                           V_6 - 5th intercostal space, left midaxillary line

6. The single channel ECG machine has one chest lead that is moved across the chest (V_1 to V_6) as each lead is recorded. A multiple channel ECG machine has six chest leads placed simultaneously on the chest. The chest lead is secured by squeezing the suction cup bulb connected to the end of the electrode. This is attached firmly to chest. If patient has large pendulous breasts, the bulbs may need to be displaced prior to electrode placement.

7. Drape all wires away from patient's chest because respirations may cause a wandering baseline

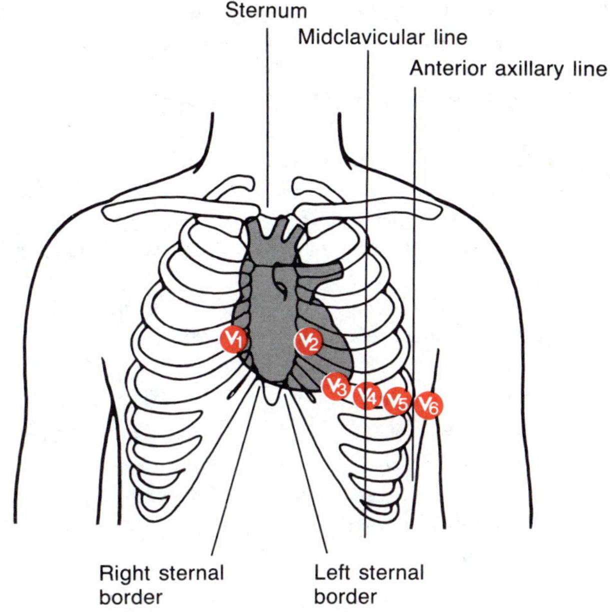

Figure 14–1 Placement of chest leads for electrocardiogram and heart sounds.

8. Set paper speed at 25 mm/sec
9. Center styles on ECG paper by turning the position control button
10. Check deflection size by pressing the ''Standardize 1mV'' button. Deflection should be set at 10 mm for 1mV or 10 small squares high on ECG paper.
11. If using a single channel machine, set lead selector at *Lead 1* and turn paper feeder on. Record approximately ten seconds of tracing. Identify lead on ECG paper. Repeat this pro-

cedure for each lead. If using a multiple channel machine, depress *auto on* button and machine automatically records and identifies each lead.

12. After recording all 12 leads, advise patient he may move as desired
13. Remove completed ECG from machine
14. Disconnect limb leads and chest electrodes from patient and turn off ECG machine
15. Wipe patient's skin with tissue or gauze to remove electrical gel
16. Label ECG recording with patient's name, medical record number, date, and time of recording

Follow-Up

1. Route ECG to appropriate physician for interpretation
2. Be prepared to begin necessary intervention
3. Make sure ECG electrodes and limb straps are cleaned to remove electrode gel

Documentation

Time of ECG
Presence of chest pain or respiratory difficulty during procedure
Primary rhythm
Dysrhythmias, if noted
Physician interpreting ECG
Patient's tolerance of procedure

SUGGESTED READING

Manzi C. Myocardial infarction. In: Robinson J, ed. Giving emergency care competently. 1st ed. Intermed Communications Inc, 1978:37.

Nursing policy and procedure manual. Dallas: Parkland Memorial Hospital, 1986: Policy # 6011-16-03.

Sumner SM, Grau PA. Guidelines for running a 12-lead EKG. Nursing 85, 1985; 15(12): 30–33.

15

PERICARDIOCENTESIS

LISA A. JONES

Purpose

To remove fluid or blood from the pericardial sac

Indications

- Cardiac tamponade (may be caused by pericarditis, trauma, acute rheumatic fever, or malignant neoplasm or lymphoma)

Contraindications

- Previous pericardial exploration

Potential Complications

- Puncture of the heart
- Arrhythmias
- Puncture of lung, stomach, or liver
- Laceration of coronary artery or myocardium
- Recurrence of tamponade

Equipment

Skin antiseptic
Local anesthetic drug
Small syringe and needle for local anesthesia
Sterile drapes and gloves

Cardiac monitor
Defibrillator
Syringe (20 ml)
Cardiac needle
Small sterile dressing

Procedure

1. Inform patient about procedure and importance of remaining immobile
2. Position patient supine with head elevated 60 degrees
3. Premedicate as ordered
4. Connect patient to cardiac monitor
5. Expose chest and prepare site with skin antiseptic
6. Drape area with sterile towels (then site is injected with local anesthetic)
7. The cardiac needle is attached to 20-ml syringe and advanced by physician until fluid is obtained. Constant suction is applied to syringe. (Pericardial fluid may be caused by trauma. Pericardial blood does not clot, while blood obtained from inadvertent puncture of one of the heart chambers does clot) (Fig. 15-1).
8. Monitor vital signs and cardiac status during procedure

Follow-Up

1. Continue to monitor cardiac status and vital signs
2. Monitor for signs of recurrent tamponade (falling blood pressure, narrowing pulse pressure, paradoxical pulse, apprehension, dyspnea, cyanosis, distended neck veins, muffled heart tones)
3. Assess for other complications such as arrhythmias

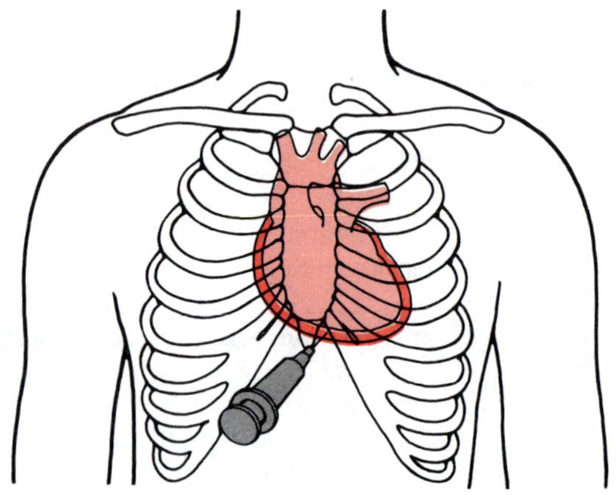

Figure 15–1 Needle placement for pericardiocentesis. Needle is advanced until fluid is obtained.

Documentation

Any visible signs of tamponade, as well as cardiac status and
   vital signs prior to procedure
Patient teaching
Allergies, medications used
Type of skin preparation
Times procedure initiated and completed
Any complications during or after procedure
Total amount and type of fluid aspirated
Cardiac status and vital signs during and after procedure
Sterile dressing applied to site

SUGGESTED READING

Baxt W, ed. Trauma-the first hour. Norwalk: Appleton-Century-Croft, 1985:121.

Brunner L, Suddarth D. The Lippincott manual of nursing practice. 1st ed. Philadelphia: JB Lippincott, 1974:243.

Sabiston D Jr, ed. Textbook of surgery. 12th ed. Philadelphia: WB Saunders, 1981:2168.

16

ROTATING TOURNIQUETS

LINDA WELD

Purpose

To decrease blood return to the heart by means of systematically applying tourniquets on the extremities

Indications

- Pulmonary edema
- Congestive heart failure

Contraindications

- Severe peripheral vascular disease
- Hypotension

Potential Complications

- Peripheral vascular insufficiency
- Hypotension

Equipment

Automatic rotating tourniquet machine
OR
Wide soft tourniquets (4)
Soft pads (4)

Procedure

1. Explain procedure
2. Position patient on back with head of bed elevated to facilitate oxygenation
3. Obtain blood pressure, and note diastolic pressure if using an automatic machine
4. Assess peripheral pulses, color, and temperature of all extremities

Automatic

5. Position machine close to patient
6. Plug machine into electrical outlet
7. Place cuffs high on appropriate extremity
8. Connect air tubes from cuffs to valves from machine
9. Close outlet valves
10. Multiply the total length of time each cuff is to be inflated times three or the number of cuffs that are to be inflated at one time, and set cuff release timer for the total number of minutes
11. Set cuff pressure with pressure control knob to just above patient's diastolic pressure
12. Turn on alarm system
13. Turn on machine
14. Open valves one at a time
15. Check arterial pulses in extremities while cuffs are inflated. If pulse is not palpable, decrease cuff pressure until pulse is palpable.
16. To obtain a blood pressure, connect tubing from the deflated cuff to a sphygmomanometer
17. To transport patient, close all valves, leave cuffs connected, turn off power to machine, disconnect from the electrical outlet, and transport patient. Never leave cuffs inflated for more than 45 minutes.

18. To discontinue therapy, close valve to cuff as a cuff deflates. Continue until all cuffs are deflated and removed.

Manual

Do procedures 1–4, then:
   5. Obtain tourniquets and pads
   6. Place pads and tourniquets high on extremities and tighten three tourniquets
   7. Check for arterial pulses in extremities below tourniquets. (If a pulse is not palpable, loosen tourniquet on that extremity until you can palpate a pulse.)
   8. After 15 minutes, loosen a tourniquet on one extremity and tighten the one on the extremity that did not previously have a tourniquet
   9. Continue to rotate tourniquets in a clockwise pattern q15min. A tourniquet should not remain tightened for more than 45 minutes.
   10. To obtain a blood pressure, place cuff on the extremity that does not have a tightened tourniquet
   11. To discontinue therapy, remove tourniquets one at a time q15min in the same pattern

Follow-Up

   1. Assess patient for signs and symptoms of heart failure as tourniquets are removed
   2. Check peripheral pulses and color and temperature of extremity

Documentation

Quality of pulses and color and temperature of extremity, prior to, during, and after procedure
Cuff pressure setting on automatic machine
Pattern of rotation if using the manual procedure

Patient's physical and psychological condition in response to procedure

SUGGESTED READING

Brunner LS, Suddarth DS. The Lippincott manual of nursing practice. 3rd ed. Philadelphia: JB Lippincott, 1982:278.

Guzetto CE, Dossey BM. Cardiovascular nursing: bodymind tapestry. Saint Louis: CV Mosby, 1984:537.

Millar S, Sampson LK, Soukup M. AACN Procedure manual for critical care. Philadelphia: WB Saunders, 1985:191.

17

THORACOTOMY

JORIE SCOTT

Purpose

To determine cause and to gain control of the major vessel and/or cardiac bleeding producing hypovolemic shock or arrest

Indications

- Hypotensive patient with blunt thoracic injury with radiologic finding of:
  - widened mediastinum
  - loss of aortic knob
  - hemothorax left apex
  - deviation of trachea or nasogastric tube
  - first or second rib fractures
  - clavicle or scapula fractures
  - anterior displacement of trachea on lateral films
  - depression of left mainstem bronchus
  - hypotensive, arrested, or prearrest patients with penetrating injuries

Contraindications

- Previous thoracotomy (because of technical problems with pleural symphysis)

Potential Complications

- Laceration of lung and heart
- Avulsion of lumbar veins and arteries
- Clamp injuries to aorta and esophagus

Equipment

Complete arrest and resuscitation equipment
Advanced cardiac life support (ACLS) drugs
Volume replacement (Ringer's lactate and blood components)
Autotransfusion setup
Cardiac monitor and defibrillator with internal and external paddles
  (pediatric or adult as indicated)
#30 French Foley with 30-ml balloon (cardiac injury)
Cardiac suture and pledgets
Betadine solution
Light source
Mask, cap, gown, and sterile gloves (various sizes)
Thoracotomy tray:
  Sterile drape
  Scalpel handle (2)
  Scalpel blade #10 and #11 (2 each)
  Needle holder (long) (4)
  Chest retractor
  Mosquitoes (6)
  Large curved Kelly clamps (4)
  Heavy curved scissors (2)
  Metsenbaum curved dissecting scissors (2)
  Tissue forceps with and without teeth (4)
  Sterile glass syringe 30 ml (2)
  Assorted needles
  Cardiac needles
  Libsehke knife and hammer

Giglii saw
Vascular clamps (2)
Rib spreaders (adult or pediatric as indicated)

Procedure

1. Establish and maintain airway, breathing, and circulation (ABCs)
2. Initiate cardiopulmonary resuscitation, if not in progress
3. Establish at least two large bore (#14 or #16 gauge) intravenous (IV) lines
4. Identify physician to be in charge of resuscitation
5. Control flow of people in room. Notify appropriate physician, respiratory therapist, radiologist, and chaplin.
6. Plug in electrical equipment—defibrillator, blood warmer, suction machine
7. Establish and maintain ongoing cardiac monitoring, and document cardiac activity
8. Administer and document ACLS drugs as indicated
9. Assist physician in preparing the chest with Betadine solution
10. Assist physician in sterile gloving
11. Direct light source to appropriate side of chest (left or right)
12. Establish sterile field and open thoracotomy tray
13. Open other supplies as needed (# 30 French Foley, cardiac suture, autotransfusion setup)
14. Connect internal defibrillator plug to defibrillator
15. Set defibrillator machine as indicated—10-20 joules/kg for adults, 2 joules/kg for pediatrics
16. Note time of chest incision
17. Note time of cardiac visualization
18. During internal cardiac massage, check for generation of a carotid pulse
19. Note time and patient's response to aortic clamping

20. Assist with defibrillation as needed
21. Note time, energy level, and patient's response to defibrillation
22. Administer volume replacement as indicated
23. Note injuries as identified in the chest
24. Notify the Operating Room of emergent case
25. Note all internal procedures done—cardiac suturing, placing of Foley into cardiac chamber for occulsion, control of other major vessel injuries, etc
26. Prepare patient for transport to Operating Room
27. Note amount of volume replacement—blood or Ringer's lactate

Follow-Up

1. Call or give prehospital and resuscitation history to appropriate nurse
2. Clothes should be labeled and sent with patient
3. Call information desk with patient disposition
4. Ensure patient's family has explanation of condition
5. Direct family to surgical waiting area
6. If patient expires:
   a) Document time code was called and physician's name
   b) Notify the medical examiner of case
   c) Notify chaplin if not done previously
   d) Prepare body for viewing for family members
   e) Prepare body for transport to medical examiner
   f) Include all documentation and clothes

Documentation

Initial assessment
Procedures performed
Therapies and patient's response

SUGGESTED READING

American College of Surgeons Committee on Trauma. Advanced trauma life support. Chicago: American College of Surgeons, 1985:73.

Baker CC, Thomas AN, Trunkey DD. The role of emergency room thoracotomy in trauma. J Trauma 1980;20:848.

Simoneau JK. Nursing process in cardiac trauma emergencies. In: Holloway N, ed. Emergency department nurses association. Core curriculum. Philadelphia: WB Saunders, 1985:43.

18

THUMPER METHOD OF AUTOMATIC RESUSCITATION

ROBERT STEELE

Purpose

To increase the effectiveness of cardiopulmonary resuscitation (CPR) by providing uniform application of chest compressions and pressure limited high-flow ventilation. Use of automatic resuscitators such as the Thumper decreases rescuers' fatigue and allows continuation of CPR efforts while transporting the patient.

Indications

- Cardiopulmonary arrest

Contraindications

Infants and children

Equipment

Thumper base plate
Compression arm-column assembly
Portable oxygen supply with two D-size (most common) or two E-size cylinders
Shoulder straps (optional)
Oxygen supply hose
Ventilation tubing
Face mask, esophageal airway, or endotracheal tube

Procedure

1. Establish manual CPR and remove any constrictive clothing
2. Position Thumper backboard under patient so that the lower part of the sternum is over center of board
3. Insert base plate into Thumper backboard. Snap the arm-column assembly into place, if unit was previously disassembled. The assembly arm should be parallel to patient (towards his feet), and not interfere with manual CPR.
4. With *all* controls in off position and the force control knob turned fully counter clockwise, connect oxygen supply source (50 psi) to oxygen inlet, which is to the left of master valve (#1)
5. Grasp piston of compressor arm just below the bottom white line, holding piston inside its housing
6. During the next manual ventilation, position compressor pad midline on lower half of sternum. Lock compressor arm in place.
7. Turn on master valve (#2), then turn cardiac compressor valve on (#2)
8. Adjust force control knob (#3) clockwise until the highest visible line on piston during compression matches the first complete drawing on the back of column, just above moveable arm assembly. Be sure to make your observations at eye level. If any partial drawing is seen, go to next complete drawing. Each marking on piston is ½ inch. Note depth of compressions.
9. Assess compressions by palpating carotid or femoral pulses. If pulses are not palpable, assess placement of compression pad and gradually adjust force control knob (#3) to increase depth of compression.

Synchronized Ventilator

1. Attach breathing hose to ventilator outlet
2. Turn ventilator switch (#4) to *On* setting

3. Adjust ventilation pressure to desired value (usually 25-30 cm H_2O) by turning ventilation pressure control (#5), during the ventilation cycle
4. Connect breathing hose to face mask, esophageal obturator airway, or endotracheal tube. Caution: If face mask is used, maintain open airway using a head-tilt or chin-lift maneuver and position mask to minimize leakage.
5. Observe the chest rise ¼ to ¾ of an inch. This may be assessed by observing piston receding into compressor arm. If ventilation is inadequate, check airway for patency and positioning, then adjust ventilation pressure control knob (#5) clockwise.
6. Ventilator may be stopped by turning ventilator switch (#4) to off setting
7. Cardiac compressions may be stopped without stopping ventilations by turning cardiac compressor knob (#2) to off position

Follow-Up

1. Continually monitor placement of compressor pad, patency of airway, generation of femoral or carotid pulse, adequacy of ventilations
2. Institute additional advanced cardiac life support procedures. Defibrillation can be performed without removing Thumper. Compressions should be stopped prior to defibrillation by turning cardiac compressor knob (#2) to off position.
3. Patient may be moved with Thumper in full operation. Special precautions should be taken to maintain proper positioning at all times.
4. If at any time Thumper becomes ineffective, manual CPR should be resumed
5. Return all controls to off position immediately following use

Documentation

Time of initiation of compressions
Location and depth of compressor pad
Character of femoral or carotid pulse
Adjustments to ventilation. Ventilation pressure and degree of rise
of chest.
Vital signs or other response to CPR

SUGGESTED READING

American Heart Association. Textbook of advanced cardiac life support. 2nd ed. Dallas: American Heart Association, 1987:41.

Babbs CF. Practical advances in cardiopulmonary resuscitation. In: Callaham ML, ed. Current therapy in emergency medicine. Toronto: BC Decker, 1987:38.

Taylor GJ, Rubin R, Tucker M, Greene HL, Rudikoff MT, Weisfeldt ML. External cardiac compression—a randomized comparison of mechanical and manual techniques. JAMA 1978;240:644–646.

NEUROLOGIC PROCEDURES

19

LUMBAR PUNCTURE

JOY A. GORZEMAN

Purpose

To obtain cerebrospinal fluid for diagnostic studies and/or for therapeutic treatment

Indications

- Differential diagnosis of central nervous system infection or subarachnoid hemorrhage
- For detecting the degree of subarachnoid block

Contraindications

- Clinical indications of increased intracranial pressure attributable to an expanding lesion (the removal of fluid may allow the lesion to expand)
- Any cutaneous or osseous infections in the lumbar area

Potential Complications

- Postpuncture headache
- Sepsis
- Herniation of the brain stem in the presence of increased intracranial pressure

Equipment

Sterile lumbar puncture tray:
 Spinal needle with stylet (adult: 20 gauge 3½″;
  pediatric: 21–22 gauge 1½″)
 Three-way stopcock
 Extension tube
 Manometer
 Syringe (3 ml) with #25 gauge 5/8″ needle
 Infiltration needle (#22 gauge 1½″)
 Specimen tubes with caps
 Antiseptic cup
 Swabs (3)
 Gauze sponges (3)
 Sterile towel
 Fenestrated drape
 Bandage

Extra spinal needle
Sterile gloves
Xylocaine (2%)
Skin antiseptic

Procedure

1. Explain to patient what procedure involves
2. Assemble and prepare equipment
3. Obtain baseline vital signs
4. Position patient on side with a pillow under the head and a pillow between knees
5. Ask patient to draw knees up to abdomen and clasp knees with hands (Fig. 19-1). Assist patient in maintaining this position by supporting him behind the knees and neck. For children, it is extremely important to hold them securely and to prevent squirming.

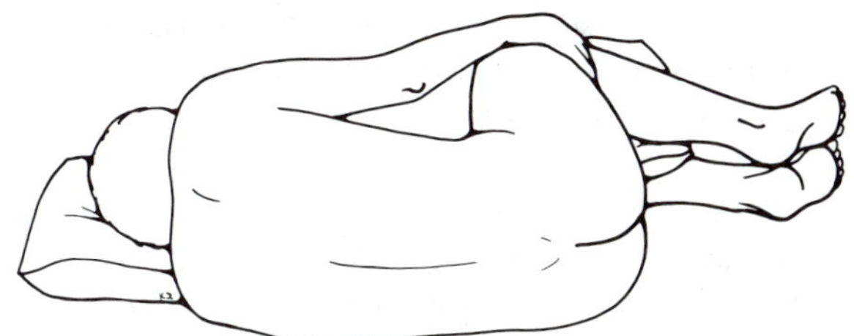

Figure 19–1 Position of patient for lumbar puncture.

6. If sitting position is preferred, have patient straddle a straight-back chair and rest head against his arms on back of chair. Or patient can sit on side of bed and lean over bedside table. For small infants, extend their arms and legs in front of them. Flex the neck so chin is almost resting on chest. Round the back by placing your thumbs on the infant's shoulders and your hands along his hips.
7. Observe infants in this position for signs of respiratory distress as the trachea is soft and can easily be obstructed when flexed
8. Help patient maintain position and remain quiet as the physician prepares the skin, injects the local anesthetic, and introduces the spinal needle
9. If pressure reading is being done, help patient slowly straighten his legs after the needle is in the subarachnoid space
10. Encourage patient to breathe quietly and not to talk
11. Three test tubes with 2–3 ml of spinal fluid in each are obtained for analysis
12. After procedure is completed, position patient on his back

Follow-Up

1. Assure that specimen tubes are labeled correctly and sent to laboratory

2. Keep patient supine 6–12 hours after procedure
3. Check vital and neurologic signs as ordered
4. Encourage fluid intake

Documentation

Appearance of spinal fluid

Number of specimens and whether or not they are sent to the
laboratory

Spinal pressure readings, if done

Vital and neurologic signs

Condition and response of patient

Medications, if given

SUGGESTED READING

Brunner LS, Suddarth DS, eds. The Lippincott manual of nursing practice.
3rd ed. Toronto: JB Lippincott, 1982:704,1169.

Miller L. Neurological assessment: a practical approach for the critical care
nurse. J Neurosurg Nurs 1979;11(1):2–5.

Rimel RW, Tyson GW. The neurologic examination in patients with central
nervous system trauma. J Neurosurg Nurs 1979;11(3):148–155.

20

SKULL TONG APPLICATION IN CERVICAL IMMOBILIZATION

KATHY GILLILAND

Purpose

To reduce and align cervical and/or high thoracic spine fractures
To provide immobilization and comfort
To assist in the prevention of further sensory or motor impairment

Indications

- Patients with unstable cervical or high thoracic spinal injuries

Contraindications

- Infants
- Paget's disease of the skull
- Massive open and/or comminuted skull fracture

Potential Complications

- Infection at pin site
- Anatomic misplacement of tong sites

Equipment

Skull tongs
Antiseptic solution (iodine, Hibiclens, Phisohex)
Antiseptic ointment (Betadine, Neosporin)

Local anesthetic (i.e., lidocaine HCl 1%)
Syringes (2–3)(5–10 ml)
Needles (3) #25 and #23 gauge
Sterile gloves
Traction setup: rope, pulley
Appropriate bed with frame, suitable for cervical traction
Razor and/or clippers
If Crutchfield tongs are used, also provide:
Small twist drill and drill bit set
Scalpel and blade
Suture

Procedure

1. Assemble all equipment
2. Prepare bed or special frame suitable for traction
3. Obtain informed consent (if applicable)
4. Obtain baseline neurologic assessment of sensory and motor function
5. Prepare insertion sites

Gardner Wells:

a) Prepare noted areas with antiseptic solution
b) Cut hair and shave if indicated per hospital routine or physician's order

Crutchfield-Vinke:

a) Prepare scalp in noted areas with antiseptic solution
b) Cut and shave hair

6. Open sterile supplies and ensure working order of drill if used for Crutchfield tongs
7. Assist in transfer of patient to bed or frame suitable for cervical traction (maintaining alignment with cervical collar)
8. Assist physician with tong insertion

Gardner Wells:

a) Prepare areas with iodine solution

b) Draw up 10 ml of anesthetic (lidocaine HCl 1%; cap with #23 gauge needle)
c) Assist with pin insertion as requested
d) Hold patient's head and neck stable during insertion

Crutchfield-Vinke:

a) Prepare areas with iodine solution
b) Draw up 10 ml anesthetic and cap with #23 gauge needle
c) Prepare scalpel and blade and hand to physician
d) Prepare small drill and drill bit
e) Assist with pin insertion as requested
f) Hold patient's head or neck stable during procedure

Follow-Up

1. Assess patient's neurologic sensory and motor function and compare to baseline
2. Clean temporal areas (etc.) to remove any drainage accumulated during insertion
3. Perform pin care to pin sites per hospital routine:
   a) ½ strength peroxide, rinse with normal saline, apply iodine ointment or Neosporin
   b) Dress Crutchfield-Vinke tong sites

Documentation

Date, time, and length of procedure; name of physician; type of tongs; and site applied

Neurologic assessment (baseline, preinsertion, patient response during insertion, and post insertion examination)

Anesthetic and analgesics used

Use of any special beds, frames, traction equipment and amount of weight applied (if weights are applied at intervals, note neurologic assessment between applications)

Patient and family teaching performed (i.e., purpose of tongs, pin care, need for fracture alignment, etc.)

SUGGESTED READING

Belland KT, Wells MA. Clinical nursing procedures. Monterey, CA: Wadsworth Health Sciences Division, 1984:288.

Hickey J. The clinical practice of neurological and neurosurgical nursing. Toronto: JB Lippincott, 1986:398.

Raimond J, Taylor JW. Neurological emergencies: effective nursing care. Rockville, MD: Aspen, 1986:30.

21

VENTRICULAR CATHETER INSERTION

KATHY GILLILAND

Purpose

To drain excess cerebrospinal fluid (CSF)

To instill irrigating solution into the ventricular system (usually antibiotics)

To provide an external drainage mechanism

To monitor intracranial pressure (ICP)

Indications

- Acute increases in ICP associated with:
  - Severe head injury or brain trauma
  - Space occupying lesions
  - Central nervous system infections
  - Brain abscesses
  - Hydrocephalus

Contraindications

- Ventricular collapse

Potential Complications

- Deterioration of neurologic status
- Rapid drainage of CSF leading to brain stem herniation
- Invasion of microorganisms leading to infection and sepsis

- Meningitis
- Catheter misplacement
- Ventricular collapse

Equipment

Hair clippers
Razor
Antiseptic scrub and solution (Betadine, Hibiclens)
Caps, masks, sterile gowns and gloves
Sterile towels
Appropriate ventricular catheter and closed external drainage
  system
Ventriculostomy tray
  Twist drill and drill bits
  Scalpel with #10 and #15 blades
  Hemostats
  Suture material
  Emesis basin
  Sterile 4×4 gauze pads
Pressure monitoring device (if monitoring ICP)

Procedure

1. Explain procedure to patient and family
2. Obtain informed consent (if applicable)
3. Assemble all equipment
4. Document baseline neurologic examination and assessment
5. Remove excess equipment and linens from bedside
6. Place patient in supine position
7. Assist in head shave, using clippers and razor as physician
   indicates (entire head or midline to frontal area)
8. Assist with 10-minute scalp preparation, using antiseptic solution
9. Assist in donning of masks, gowns, and gloves

10. Open sterile supplies
11. Hold patient's head (if needed) in midline position
12. Assist as physician:
    a) Performs another preparation with antiseptic solution
    b) Makes scalp incision with #10 blade
    c) Uses twist drill to make burr hole in skull
    d) Prepares to enter catheter into tissues
    e) Advances catheter through a stylet into lateral ventricle's anterior horn or occipital horn
    f) Attaches catheter to drainage system
    g) Sutures catheter in place
    h) Applies firm contained sterile dressing
13. Offer patient support as needed throughout procedure
14. Ensure catheter is secured, and a sterile contained dressing is applied

Follow-Up

1. Clean patient environment
2. Perform follow-up neurologic assessment (q15min $\times$ 4, q30min $\times$ 2, then q1h $\times$ 4)

Documentation

Procedure performed including: physician's name, date, time and length of procedure, type of drain, and system used

Neurologic assessment during and after procedure with comparison to preprocedure examination

Note anesthetics or analgesics used, before, during, and after procedure

Amount, color, and odor of fluid drained

Patient and/or family teaching regarding procedure and use of catheter

ICPs, if a monitoring system is used

SUGGESTED READING

Hickey J. The clinical practice of neurological and neurosurgical nursing. Toronto: JB Lippincott, 1986:273.

Raimond J, Taylor JW. Neurological emergencies: effective nursing care. Rockville, MD: Aspen, 1986:146.

Rudy E. Advanced neurological and neurosurgical nursing. Saint Louis: CV Mosby, 1984:133.

GASTROINTESTINAL AND GENITOURINARY PROCEDURES

22

ENEMA

BARBARA KALO

Purpose

To evacuate lower bowel

To instill medication or a soothing agent into rectum

To prepare lower bowel for diagnostic and/or operative procedure

Indications

- Constipation or fecal impaction
- Instillation of medication (locally)

Contraindications

- Trauma to bowel
- Recent lower bowel surgery

Potential Complications

- Increased distention of walls of lower bowel, if air is introduced with enema solution

- Spasm of intestinal wall with rapid introduction of fluid
- Perforation of rectum

Equipment

Enema solution
Enema bag and tubing
Bath thermometer
Water-soluble lubricant
Disposable gloves
Bedpan
Toilet tissue

Procedure

1. Gather equipment and prepare solution as ordered
2. The amount of solution should be 700–1,000 ml at 37 °C, unless otherwise ordered
3. Identify patient
4. Explain procedure to patient
5. Provide privacy
6. Position patient on left side with knees flexed. Other positions may be dorsal recumbent or knee-chest.
7. Drape patient, and don nonsterile gloves
8. Expel air from tubing by running solution to tip of the catheter before insertion
9. Lubricate 2–3 inches of rectal tube
10. Insert lubricated tube approximately 4 inches into rectum
11. Solution container should be raised no higher than 18 inches above level of patient
12. Slowly administer as much of the fluid as patient can comfortably tolerate
13. If patient experiences abdominal pain or cramping, instruct patient to take deep breaths, clamp tubing for a few seconds if necessary, and then resume instillation of fluid

14. Clamp tube after administration of fluid to prevent air from entering lower bowel
15. Remove tube
16. Encourage patient to retain solution for 5–10 minutes. If retention enema, solution should be retained for as long as possible.
17. Assist patient onto bedpan or to bathroom
18. Have toilet tissue and callbell within patient's reach
19. Instruct patient to call when enema is expelled and not to flush toilet so that results can be noted by nurse

Follow-Up

1. Assist patient off bedpan and/or back into bed
2. Clean equipment
3. Assess comfort of patient
4. Note amount and color of solution returned
5. Note any abnormal findings such as pus, mucus, blood, or worms
6. Observe stool for color and consistency
7. Observe for expulsion of flatus
8. Note if desired effects (such as sedation) were obtained
9. Report results to doctor

Documentation

Date and time of procedure
Type and amount of solution
Results
Patient's tolerance to procedure
Instructions to patient and/or family as necessary

SUGGESTED READING

Brunner LS, Suddarth DS. The Lippincott manual of nursing practice. 3rd ed. Philadelphia: JB Lippincott, 1982:415.

King EM, Wieck L, Dyer M. Illustrated manual of nursing techniques. 1st ed. New York: JB Lippincott, 1977:144.

The nursing policy and procedure manual. Dallas: Parkland Memorial Hospital, 1987. Policy #6011-30-02.

23

GASTRIC LAVAGE

BARBARA KALO

Purpose

To administer and siphon back solution from the stomach

Indications

- Poisoning
- Gastrointestinal bleeding
- Diagnostic studies of stomach
- Preparation for surgery

Contraindications

- Insertion of tube nasally if fracture present
- Ingestion of strong alkalis
- Ingestion of strychnine (stimulation of nasogastric tube may trigger convulsions)

Potential Complications

- Damage to mucous membrane of gastrointestinal tract
- Gastric distention
- Electrolyte imbalance
- Hypothermia, if using iced saline
- Chills
- Bradycardia
- Aspiration

Equipment

Large bore nasogastric (NG) tube
Water-soluble lubricant
Aspirating syringe
Tape
Stethoscope
Unsterile gloves
Emesis basin
Glass of water with a straw
Bath towel
Irrigating solution or antidote as ordered
Container for irrigating solution
Tubing with Y-connector
Hemostat or clamp for tubing
Container for stomach content returns
Available suction

Procedure

1. Gather equipment
2. Identify patient
3. Explain procedure to patient
4. Wash hands
5. Place towel under chin and over chest of patient
6. Measure length of NG tube by placing tip of tube to earlobe, then running length of NG tube to bridge of nose, and to xiphoid process. Mark tube with tape.
7. Don unsterile gloves
8. Lubricate approximately 6–8 inches of NG tube
9. With patient in sitting position, insert NG tube to back of nose and throat. Have patient flex head forward and instruct to swallow as tube is advanced smoothly to the marking.
10. To assure proper placement, aspirate gastric contents and auscultate with stethoscope over gastric area while inserting

30–50 ml of air into NG tube. If gastric contents are not aspirated or insertion of air cannot be auscultated over the gastric area, reposition tube.
11. Tape NG tube in place
12. Instill saline, 100–200 ml at a time and then aspirate with large irrigating syringe (or by gravity) into a container
13. Iced saline is used to control gastric bleeding
14. Repeat procedure until solution returns clear

Follow-Up

1. Assess patient for any complications
2. Obtain specimen for laboratory analysis
3. Assess comfort of patient
4. Clean equipment
5. Note character of stomach returns

Documentation

Date and time of procedure
Type and amount of irrigating solution
Disposition of specimen
Character of stomach content returns
Patient's tolerance to procedure
Instructions to patient and/or family as necessary

SUGGESTED READING

King EM, Wieck L, Dyer M. Illustrated manual of nursing techniques. New York: JB Lippincott, 1977:159.

Lewis SM, Collier IC. Medical-surgical nursing: assessment and management of clinical problems. New York: McGraw Hill, 1982:943, 1657.

Fugleberg BB, Brogdon E, Mossing K, Tabor B. Management of upper gastrointestinal hemorrhage. In: Millar S, Sampson LK, Soukup SM. AACN procedure manual for critical care. Philadelphia: WB Saunders, 1985:363.

Nursing policy and procedure manual. Dallas: Parkland Memorial Hospital, 1987. Policy #6011-30-04.

Tandberg D, Troutman W. Gastric lavage in the poisoned patient. In: Roberts JR, Hedges JR, eds. Clinical procedures in emergency medicine. 1st ed. Philadelphia: WB Saunders, 1985:762.

24

NASOGASTRIC INTUBATION

BARBARA CLARK MIMS

Purpose

To empty stomach contents
To assess guaiac and pH of stomach contents
To lavage stomach
To instill medications into stomach
To administer feedings into stomach

Indications

- Gastrointestinal bleed
- Drug overdose

Contraindications

- Facial fractures
- Patients who have had surgery on esophagus or stomach (physician should insert)

Potential Complications

- Nasal mucosa erosion
- Trauma to gastric mucosa
- Reflux esophagitis
- Bradycardia
- Hyperventilation

Equipment

Nasogastric (NG) tube
Water-soluble lubricant
Irrigating syringe (50 ml)
1-inch adhesive tape
Emesis basin
Suction source
Stethoscope

Procedure

1. Identify patient, provide privacy, and explain procedure, if feasible
2. Position patient in a comfortable sitting or recumbent position with head slightly flexed
3. Measure length of NG tube to be inserted by placing tip of NG tube at earlobe, then running the length of the NG tube to nose, and then to xiphoid process. Mark this point with a piece of tape (Fig. 24–1).
4. Apply small amount of water-soluble lubricant to NG tube
5. Insert tube:
   a) Pass NG tube gently into nasopharynx. NG tube should be inserted along medial floor of nose initially and then toward ipsilateral earlobe. The NG tube may have to be slightly rotated to move it from the nose to the pharyngeal area.
   b) When pharyngeal area is reached, encourage patient to swallow. Offer sips of water if necessary to the alert patient.
   c) In intubated patient, passage of NG tube may be facilitated by flexing patient's head on his chest
   d) Insert NG tube until premeasured length is reached. Keep emesis basin handy in case patient vomits.
   e) If respiratory distress is noted, withdraw NG tube immedi-

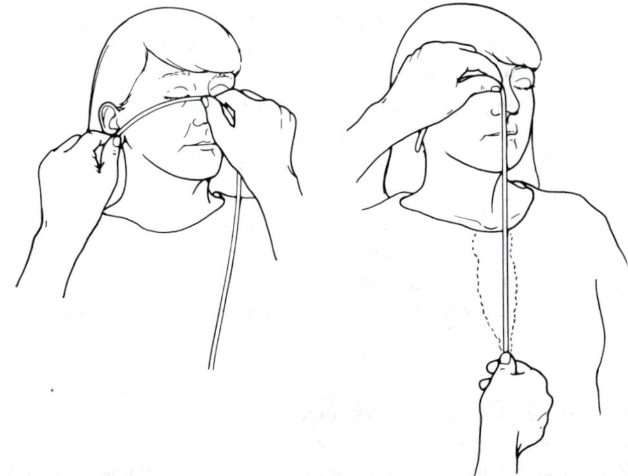

Figure 24–1 Measuring length of tube to be inserted for nasogastric intubation (from earlobe to nose to xiphoid process).

ately. This may indicate placement in trachea or bronchus.
  f) Verify placement of NG tube in stomach by aspirating gastric contents (using irrigation syringe) or by injecting 10–20 ml air into tube while listening over stomach with stethoscope for *rush* of air
  g) Tape NG tube in place with 1-inch adhesive tape using butterfly technique (spiraling the wings down the tube)
6. Attach to low gomco or low wall suction (40–60 mm Hg), if ordered by physician. Salem sump tubes require continuous suction. NG tubes without air vents, such as Levine tubes, require intermittent suction, however, these are rarely used.

Follow-Up

1. Clean patient and provide comfort measures as indicated

2. If patient is ambulatory, secure NG tube to patient gown using a rubber band and safety pin to prevent tugging on NG tube when patient ambulates
3. Maintain patency of NG tube by irrigating and repositioning NG tube as necessary. **CAUTION:** When the patient has undergone gastric or esophageal surgery, the nurse should *never* reposition or remove the NG tube.
4. Observe color and consistency of NG drainage
5. Record intake and output carefully
6. Restrain patient as needed to prevent removal of NG tube. (This requires physician's order in some institutions.)

Documentation

Record size and type of NG tube, amount and type of suction, and name of person inserting NG tube

Record color and pertinent characteristics (pH, guaiac, etc.) of aspirate

Record patient's tolerance of procedure

SUGGESTED READING

Barrett JE. Inserting and removing a nasogastric tube. Nursing 1984;7:8L–8V.

Millar S, Sampson LK, Soukup M. AACN procedure manual for critical care. Philadelphia: WB Saunders, 1985:363.

Persons CB. Critical care procedures and protocols. A nursing process approach. Philadelphia: JB Lippincott, 1987:194.

Smith S, Duell D. Clinical nursing skills. Los Altos: National Nursing Review, 1985:360.

25

PARACENTESIS

LISA A. JONES

Purpose

To remove accumulated fluid from abdominal cavity (a needle paracentesis can be done to detect intra-abdominal hemorrhage attributable to abdominal trauma)

Indications

- Ascites
- Suspected intra-abdominal hemorrhage attributable to abdominal trauma

Contraindications

- Gunshot wound to abdomen
- Obstructed or distended loops of bowel

Potential Complications

- Infection
- Bleeding attributable to vessel trauma
- Penetration of bowel
- Shock and hypovolemia due to fluid shifts from the general circulation to the abdomen in attempt to replace fluid removed
- Puncture of urinary bladder
- Mesenteric or rectus sheath hematoma

Equipment

Skin antiseptic
Sterile drapes and gloves
Small needle and syringe for local anesthetic
Local anesthetic drug
Large bore, short beveled spinal needle
Syringe
Three-way stopcock
Sterile tubing
Sterile specimen container
Small sterile dressing

Procedure

1. Inform patient of procedure
2. Have patient empty bladder
3. Position patient in Fowler's position
4. Expose, cleanse, and drape abdomen
5. Local anesthetic is administered
6. Needle paracentesis is done with patient in supine position. Needle is connected to syringe and suction is applied as needle is advanced slowly into the abdomen in four quadrants. Return of nonclotting blood is a positive result.
7. For removal of large accumulations of peritoneal fluid, a three-way stopcock is attached between needle and syringe with sterile tubing connected to the other end of the stopcock. The tubing is connected to a sterile container.
8. Needle (intravenous catheter may be used with needle removed after insertion, and catheter left in place) is then advanced by physician below the umbilicus, with suction applied to syringe, until fluid is obtained
9. The stopcock is then turned open to the tubing, and fluid is slowly drained into the container, which is placed below patient

10. Observe patient during procedure for pallor, cyanosis, syncope, and other signs of shock, as well as pulse and respiratory status
11. Apply dressing when catheter is removed

Follow-Up

1. Place patient in comfortable position
2. Record amount and kind of fluid removed
3. Monitor patient's vital signs frequently
4. Notify Operating Room if patient has a positive needle paracentesis because surgery is necessary to locate and repair injury

Documentation

Patient and family teaching done
Type of skin preparation and anesthetic
Total amount, color, and character of fluid removed
Any complications during procedure
Vital signs following procedure
Any complications following procedure
Sterile dressings applied to site
Results of needle paracentesis

SUGGESTED READING

Brunner L, Suddarth D, eds. The Lippincott manual of nursing practice. 4th ed. Philadelphia: JB Lippincott, 1986:437.

Luckman J, Sorenson K. Medical-surgical nursing. Philadelphia: WB Saunders, 1974:1121.

Sabiston D Jr. ed. Textbook of surgery. 12th ed. Philadelphia: WB Saunders, 1981:378.

Shires GT. Care of the trauma patient. New York: McGraw Hill, 1979:293.

26

PERITONEAL LAVAGE

JORIE SCOTT

Purpose

To evaluate the intra-abdominal space of patients who have sustained blunt abdominal trauma (quickly, inexpensively, and in a relatively simple safe surgical procedure)

To diagnose adult intra-abdominal injury and possibly to provide the first clue to biliary or intestinal injury

Indications

- Patients who have a history of blunt abdominal trauma and who have altered pain response—head injury, alcohol or drug overlay, or spinal cord trauma
- Unexplained hypovolemia following multiple trauma
- Suspected intra-abdominal injury associated with low rib fractures or trauma of the lower chest, flank, or buttocks
- Carefully selected patients with penetrating trauma (to avoid false positive results, a supraumbilical approach may be employed with pelvic fractures)

Contraindications

- History of multiple abdominal operations
- Obvious indications for exploratory laparotomy—free air, peritonitis
- Penetrating trauma
- Gravid uterus in third trimester

Potential Complications

- Abdominal wall bleeding producing a false positive result
- Visceral damage
- Perforating of intra-abdominal injury
- Peritonitis

Equipment

Betadine solution
4 × 4 gauze sponges
Gown, gloves, mask, caps for two
Lidocaine 1% with epinephrine
Preparation blade (weck blade, razor)
3-inch tape
Laboratory specimen tubes
Sedation (if indicated)
Light source
Peritoneal lavage catheter (adult or pediatric as indicated)
Ringer's lactate 500 ml or 100 ml (as indicated for pediatric
    patients—10 ml/kg)
Intravenous (IV) tubing
Peritoneal lavage tray
Syringes (2) (10 ml)
#25 gauge 1-inch needle (2)
#18 gauge 1-inch needle (2)
Sterile towels
Scalpel and handle with #10 and #11 blades
Tissue forceps (2)
Allis clips (4)
Hemostats (6)
Closing suture material
Equipment to place nasogastric (NG) tube (if not in place)
Equipment to place Foley catheter (if not in place)

Procedure

1. Maintain patient's airway, breathing, and circulation (ABCs)
2. Obtain baseline vital signs
3. Explain procedure to patient and family
4. Determine if patient is allergic to Betadine
5. Place NG tube to low gomco suction to decompress stomach
6. Place Foley catheter to decompress bladder
7. Administer sedation, if patient is extremely combative or for some pediatric cases
8. Restrain patient, if indicated (for example patients with altered mental status who are unable to cooperate)
9. Assist physician in preparing abdominal margin to pubic area, flank to flank
10. Assist physician in anesthetizing skin
11. Direct light source
12. Open peritoneal lavage tray to establish sterile field
13. Assist physician with cap, mask, gown, and gloves
14. Open peritoneal lavage catheter onto sterile field
15. Open closing suture onto sterile field
16. Set up Ringer's lactate solution, keep end of IV tubing sterile
17. Assist physician with insertion of catheter (Fig. 26–1)
18. Note and document syringe aspirate of lavage catheter
19. If grossly bloody aspirate, prepare patient and family for surgical procedure
20. If no grossly bloody aspirate, assist physician in connecting IV tubing to peritoneal lavage catheter
21. Infuse Ringer's lactate at a wide open rate
22. Allow fluid to remain in abdomen 5–10 minutes after solution is infused
23. Lower Ringer's lactate bag to below level of abdomen. This siphons the fluid over 20–30 minutes.
24. If fluid is not returning freely, notify physician

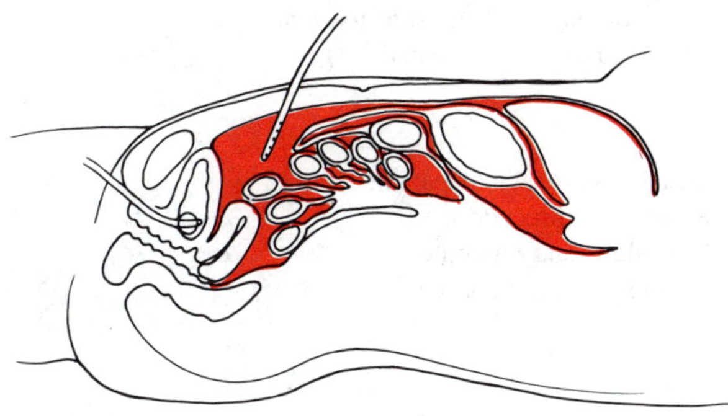

Figure 26–1 Catheter placement during peritoneal lavage.

25. When fluid returns, send lavage specimens as ordered. Positive findings are as follows:

Erythrocyte count (unspun)	100,000/cm
White cell count	5,000/cm
Gram stain for bacteria	+
Smear for vegetable fiber	+
Spun hematocrit	2

26. Monitor ABCs and vital signs before and after procedure
27. Assist physician in closing abdomen
28. Assist in placing sterile dressing to abdomen

Follow-Up

If positive findings:
1. Assist physician in obtaining operating permit
2. Assure Operating Room notified
3. Notify family of findings

If negative findings:
1. Prepare patient for admission to hospital for observation
2. Notify family

3. Continue with head-to-toe evaluation
4. Intervene as indicated

Documentation

Initial assessment of patient
Reason for procedure
Procedure and outcome
Ongoing assessment

SUGGESTED READING

American College of Surgeons Committee on Trauma. Advanced trauma life support. Chicago: American College of Surgeons, 1985:5.

Knezevich B. Nursing process in abdominal trauma. In: Holloway NM, ed. Emergency department nurses association. Core curriculum. Philadelphia: WB Saunders, 1985:5.

Urosevich PR, ed. Nursing photobook. Dealing with emergencies. Horsham, PA: Intermed Communications 1980:84.

27

URETHRAL CATHETERIZATION

MOLLY A. SEAMAN

Purpose

To provide continuous bladder drainage

Indications

- Urinary retention
- To monitor urinary output accurately
- Patients without bladder control
- Patients going to surgery
- Multiple trauma patients

Contraindications

- Urethral injuries
- Patients able to void by themselves

Potential Complications

- Infections
- Urethral trauma
- Urinary retention

Equipment

Sterile urinary catheter
Catheterization tray:
    Sterile collection bag (urimeter optional)

Syringe (10 ml) and sterile water (10 ml)
Lubricant
Povidone-iodine solution and cotton balls
Sterile gloves and drapes

Procedure

1. Gather equipment at bedside
2. If patient is awake, explain all procedures carefully
3. Provide comfortable and private area for patient
4. Assist patient to dorsal recumbent position (if not contraindicated), and drape with a top sheet
5. Open equipment and place onto sterile field. Place pad under patient.
6. Put on sterile gloves, and place a fenestrated drape over perineum
7. Pour povidone-iodine solution onto cotton balls
8. Test balloon by inflating with sterile water, then deflate
9. Squeeze lubricant onto tray to lubricate catheter tip
10. Female patients—locate meatus by separating labia minora. Cleanse meatus and folds of labia with the other hand. Use downward stroke with cotton ball and discard. Cleanse with at least three cotton balls (Fig.27–1).
11. Male patients—lift penis upward. Cleanse meatus of urethra, using circular motion. Use sponge once and discard. Uncircumcised males should have the foreskin retracted to cleanse adequately.
12. Insert catheter into urethra until urine begins to flow. Insert about 1–2 inches more to ensure urethra is passed.
13. Then inflate balloon with sterile water. Gently pull back until resistance is met.
14. Connect catheter to connecting tubing, if not already done
15. Tape catheter to patient's leg. Assure there is no tension on catheter.

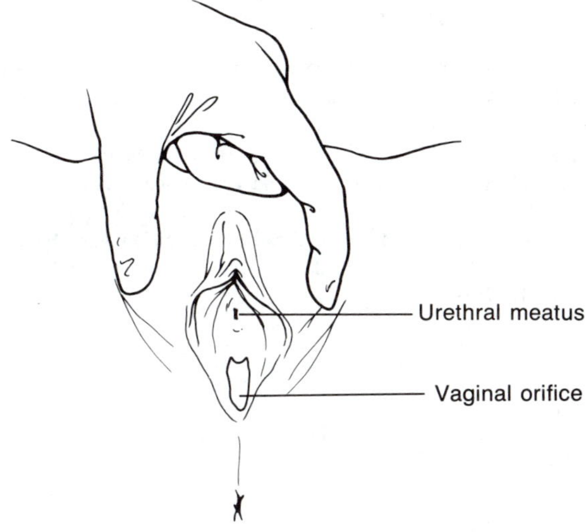

Figure 27–1 Urethral catheterization for the female. Locate meatus by separating labia minora.

16. Secure bag to side of bed or stretcher

Follow-Up

1. Note color and amount of drainage
2. Check bladder to assure no distention
3. Continue to monitor drainage

Documentation

Size of catheter, and amount of urine output
Any difficulty encountered, and if physician notified
Intake and output until catheter removed

SUGGESTED READING

Baily JA, Dupont J, Gryetvan M, O'Brien P, et al. Abdominal pelvic emergencies. In: Robinson J, ed. Dealing with emergencies. Horsham, PA: Intermed Communication, 1980:86.

Dugas BW. The care of patients who have urinary problems. In: Dugas BW, ed. Introduction to patient care. 2nd ed. Philadelphia: WB Saunders, 1972:390.

King EM, Wieck L, Dyer M. Urethral catheterization. In: King EM, Dyer M, Wieck L, eds. Illustrated manual of nursing techniques. New York: JB Lippincott, 1977:64.

OBSTETRICAL AND GYNECOLOGIC PROCEDURES

28

CULDOCENTESIS

PAMELA Y. DONNELLY
PAULA K. OVENS

Purpose

To evaluate fluid in the intraperitoneal space in order to diagnose suspected ectopic pregnancies, suspected ovarian cysts, and pelvic inflammatory disease. The procedure involves insertion of a hollow needle through the posterior vaginal wall into the retroperitoneal space (Pouch of Douglas) where a specimen of fluid can be aspirated.

Indications

- To determine the origin of acute lower abdominal pain in adult females

Contraindications

- Pelvic mass (e.g., tubo-ovarian abscess, appendiceal abscess, ovarian mass)
- Nonmobile retroverted uterus
- Coagulopathies
- Previous salpingitis
- Pelvic peritonitis

Potential Complications

- Rupture of an undiagnosed tubo-ovarian abscess
- Perforation of the bowel or an undiagnosed pelvic kidney
- Bleeding from the insertion site in women with clotting disorders

Equipment

Stethoscope
Sphygmomanometer
Sterile gloves
Vaginal speculum
Tenaculum
Syringe (20ml)
#20 or #22 gauge spinal needle
Syringe (10ml) with #22 gauge needle (optional)
Lidocaine 1% (10ml) (optional)

Procedure

1. Take complete set of vital signs
2. Advise patient of procedure and what to expect
3. Ready examination room. Assemble equipment as indicated. The physician may wish to provide a local anesthetic injection prior to culdocentesis.
4. Place patient in lithotomy position with head of table slightly elevated and both feet secured in stirrups
5. Assist physician with procedure, which involves:
   a) A bimanual examination to confirm size and position of uterus and absence of a pelvic mass
   b) Insertion of vaginal speculum to ascertain adequate exposure of posterior lip of the cervix
   c) Applying tenaculum to pull the cervix toward the symphysis
   d) Anesthetizing puncture site with 1% lidocaine (optional)

   e) Positioning spinal needle in the vaginal wall, penetrating the site 2 to 2½ cm, then slowly withdrawing and applying suction on the syringe simutaneously taking care not to aspirate any accumulated blood in the vagina (Fig. 28–1)

   f) Removing speculum from the vagina

6. Assist patient into a comfortable desired position

Follow-Up

1. Repeat patient's vital signs q15min
2. Observe for increasing lower abdominal pain
3. Observe for bleeding at insertion site (i.e., vaginal bleeding)
4. Continual assessment of hemodynamic status

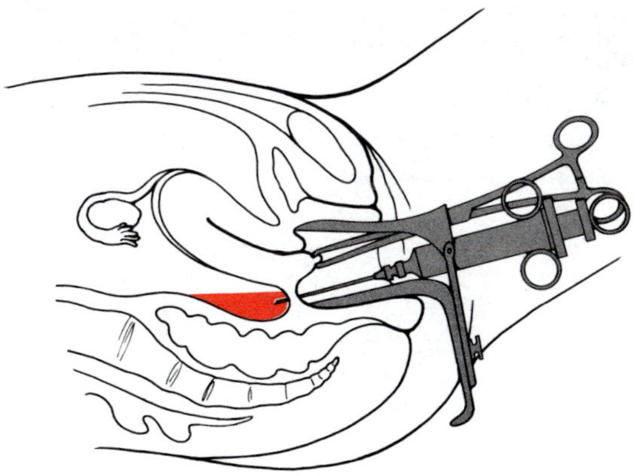

Figure 28–1   Aspiration of fluid from retroperitoneal space.

Documentation

Patient's response to procedure
Medical findings from culdocentesis
Vital signs
Vaginal bleeding
Planned medical intervention(s)

SUGGESTED READING

Main M, Main EK. Obstetrics & gynecology. Chicago: Year Book Medical Publishers, 1984:130.

Pritchard JA, MacDonald PC, Gant NF. Williams obstetrics. 17th ed. Norwalk, CT: Appleton-Century-Crofts, 1985:423.

Roberts JR, Hedges JR, eds. Clinical procedures in emergency medicine. Philadelphia: WB Saunders, 1985: 740.

29

DILATATION AND CURETTAGE

PAMELA Y. DONNELLY
PAULA K. OVENS

Purpose

To evaluate abnormal uterine bleeding as a diagnostic and/or therapeutic procedure

Indications

- First trimester abortions
- Dysfunctional uterine bleeding
- Dysmenorrhea
- Endometrial cancer

Contraindications

- Viable fetus
- Hemodynamically unstable patient

Potential Complications

- Uterine perforation
- Cervical laceration
- Hemorrhage
- Incomplete removal of fetus and placenta
- Sepsis

Equipment

Stethoscope
Sphygmomanometer
Sterile vaginal preparation equipment
#18 gauge intravenous catheter
Sterile gown and gloves
Sterile dilatation and curettage (D&C) instrument set:
  Large speculum
  Tenaculum
  Curette (small, medium, and large)
  Uterine sound
  Cervical dilators
Vacuum-suction machine set (optional):
  Vacuum machine
  Vacuum tubing
  Curettes (8mm, 10mm, and 12mm)

Procedure

1. Obtain history and physical assessment, including gravidity, parity, abortions, last menstrual period, abdominal pain, time of onset and amount of vaginal bleeding, and tissue passed
2. Provide psychological and emotional support
3. Take a complete set of vital signs including a tilt test. The tilt test is used to evaluate the patient's hemodynamic status. Take both blood pressure and pulse with patient lying in supine position. Then, change patient's position to sitting or standing. A change of 20 mm Hg or more in systolic or diastolic pressure and/or an increase or decrease of more than 20 beats per minute is considered a positive tilt test. Patients with a positive test should be evaluated for hypovolemia.
4. Draw laboratory tests as ordered by the physician, such as complete blood count and urine analysis. A type and cross

for blood may be needed if the patient's circulating blood volume is decreased.

5. Start intravenous infusion (IV) with #8 gauge or larger needle. If ordered, pitocin or oxytocin may be added to the fluid.
6. Confirm that an operative permit has been obtained for this procedure
7. Place patient in lithotomy position with the head slightly elevated and both feet secured in stirrups. Save all tissue passed from patient's uterus. Endometrial tissue and/or products of conception should be evaluated by pathology.
8. Do a sterile vaginal preparation as outlined in *Sterile Vaginal Preparation* procedure
9. Repeat patient's vital signs and prepare equipment in room. (Sterile gown and gloves for physician, sterile D&C instrument set, and vacuum-suction machine set [optional].)
10. Prepare and administer narcotics as ordered (a paracervical block may be used)
11. Advise patient of the noise the vacuum-suction machine makes, so as not to startle patient
12. Assist physician with procedure, which involves:
    a) A bimanual examination for size and position of uterus
    b) Insertion of a vaginal speculum to ascertain adequate exposure of cervix
    c) Applying tenaculum to the anterior lip of the cervix
    d) Assessing size of uterus by inserting a uterine sound
    e) Dilating cervix with cervical dilators
    f) Removing products of conception with curettes or vacuum aspiration
    g) Remove speculum from vagina
13. Assist patient into a comfortable position

Follow-up

1. Repeat patient's vital signs q15min ×4, then q30min ×2

2. As patient awakens, assess progress with respect to vaginal bleeding and pain
3. Repeat hematocrit as ordered by physician
4. Send all tissue to laboratory to be evaluated by pathology
5. Provide discharge instructions:
   a) Use of sanitary pads only - no tampons - for 1 week
   b) *No* intercourse for 1 week.
   c) Take no tub baths or douches for 1 week. Showers are recommended.
   d) Take temperature each morning and night for 1 week. If temperature is over 100.4°F, consult physician.
   e) Vaginal bleeding may not be present for 2-3 days following a dilatation and curettage. It may then begin like a normal period for 7-10 days. A few women do not bleed at all following this procedure, which is normal for them.
   f) Next normal period should begin in 4-8 weeks. It is possible to get pregnant before first period. Therefore, if pregnancy is not desired, use the means of birth control suggested by physician.

Documentation

Beginning and ending time of procedure
Patient's response
Amount of vaginal bleeding
Medical finding
Vital signs
Medications administered for procedure
Discharge instructions

SUGGESTED READING

Benson RC, ed. Handbook of obstetrics and gynecology. 8th ed. Los Altos,

CA: Lange Medical Publications, 1983:439.

Mishell DR Jr. Family planning. In: Berkow R, ed. The Merk manual. 14th ed. Rahway, NJ: Merk Sharp & Dohme Research Laboratories, 1982:1699.

Pritchard JA, MacDonald PC, Grant NF. Williams obstetrics. 17th ed. Norwalk, CT: Appleton-Century-Croft, 1985:423.

30

PRECIPITOUS DELIVERY

PAMELA Y. DONNELLY
PAULA K. OVENS

Purpose

To control vaginal delivery precipitated by rapid labor

Indications

- Rapid cervical dilatation and effacement

Contraindications

- None

Potential Complications

- Lacerations of the cervix, vagina, vulva, or perineum
- Postpartum hemorrhage
- Amniotic fluid embolism
- Newborn intracranial trauma

Equipment

Sterile gloves
Bulb syringe
Absorbable towel
Clamps (peons) (2)
Bandage scissors
Baby blanket

Procedure

1. Provide reassurance to patient and/or family member(s)
2. Place the patient in lithotomy position with the head slightly elevated and both feet secured in stirrups
3. Remove bulb syringe and towel from package
4. Don sterile gloves
5. With towel, support baby's head with one hand, applying gentle pressure to the head to prevent sudden expulsion and undue stretching of perineum or brain damage to infant
6. After infant's head is delivered, wipe face quickly and aspirate nares and mouth with the bulb syringe
7. Next, pass your fingers to the neck of the infant to ascertain whether it is encircled by the umbilical cord. If a coil is felt, draw cord down between the fingers and, if loose enough, slip it over the head. If it is applied too tightly, it should be clamped with two clamps and cut.
8. Delivery of the shoulders occurs following spontaneous external rotation. The sides of the head are grasped with two hands and gentle downward traction applied until the anterior shoulder appears under the pubic arch (Fig. 30-1).
9. Then, by an upward movement of the head, the posterior shoulder is delivered
10. The rest of the body slides out easily, usually with a gush of amniotic fluid
11. Once infant is born, hold it with its head slightly lower than its body to promote drainage of mucous
12. Suction mouth and nose of the infant again with bulb syringe
13. Clamp umbilical cord with two peons and cut
14. Dry infant to prevent heat loss
15. Wrap the baby in a warm blanket and place on mother's abdomen to provide warmth

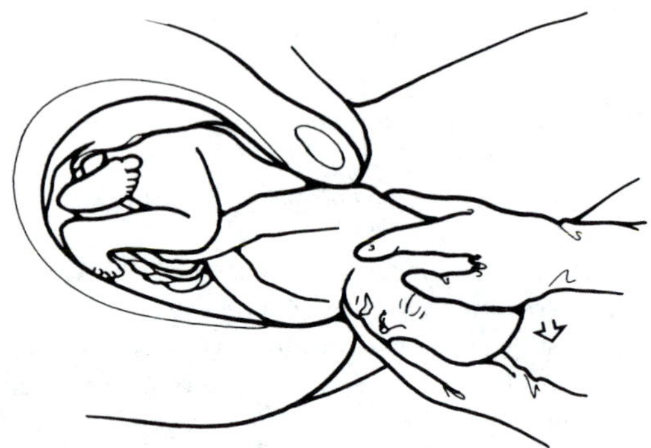

Figure 30–1 Apply downward pressure to deliver anterior shoulder during precipitous delivery.

Follow-Up

1. Observe infant's respiratory status to ensure an open and patent airway
2. Observe for signs of placental separation, which can be detected by a gush of blood from the vaginal opening and further protrusion of the umbilical cord
3. Monitor maternal vital signs
4. Provide continuous fundal massage (after placenta delivered) to ensure firm uterine tone, thus preventing postpartum hemorrhage

Documentation

Time of delivery of infant and placenta
Maternal and infant status
Maternal-infant attachment behaviors

SUGGESTED READING

Benson RC. Handbook of obstetrics and gynecology. 8th ed. Los Altos, CA: Lange Medical Publications, 1983:465.

Dilts PV Jr. Physiology and management of normal pregnancy. In: Berkow RE, ed. The Merk manual. 14th ed. Rahway, NJ: Merk Sharp & Dohme Research Laboratories, 1982:1713.

Jenson MD, Benson RD, Bobak IN. Maternity care: a nurse and the family. Saint Louis: CV Mosby, 1981:339.

Main DM, Main EK. Obstetrics and gynecology. Chicago: Year Book Medical Publishers, 1984:94.

Pritchard JA, MacDonald PC, Grant NF. Williams obstetrics. 17th ed. Norwalk, CT: Appleton-Century-Crofts, 1985:331.

31

EXAMINATION OF SEXUALLY ASSAULTED PATIENT

NANCY WEINBERG

Purpose

To meet physiologic and psychological needs of the patient
To reduce the sexually assaulted victim's stress
To preserve evidence
To provide notification of authorities, family, and friends

Indications

- Alleged sexual assault

Contraindications

- None

Potential Complications

- Possible psychological complications

Equipment

Rape kit
Speculum
Anascope
White sheet
Red top blood laboratory tube
Tourniquet

Venapuncture needle and jacket
Bandage
Gonorrhea culture bottle (3)
Microscopic slide (3)
Microscopic slide cover slip (3)

Procedure

1. Initial crisis intervention
2. Immediately provide privacy for sexually assaulted patient
3. Registration of sexually assaulted patient may be completed in privacy of examination room or private waiting area
4. Primary nursing is the recommended model for providing care to sexually assaulted patient
5. Assess vital signs (temperature, heart rate, respiratory rate, and blood pressure)
6. Obtain brief history from patient, include areas of penetration (vaginal, oral, and anal)
7. Obtain written informed consent for examination and treatment. The informed consent must include explanation of the following phases of examination and evidence collected:
   a) Medical and gynecologic history
   b) Physical examination
   c) Collection of evidence
   d) Photographs, if indicated
   e) Release of information to legal authorities
   f) Treatment rendered
8. Instruct patient not to urinate, defecate, or wash genital area until after evidence is collected. Also instruct patient not to drink anything if oral penetration was involved in assault.
9. Advise patient of readily available support and counseling services, such as Rape Victim Advocates or Rape Crisis Workers. Ask patient if she (he) would like you to notify the services so they may provide additional support and expertise in counseling.

10. Once the seal is broken on the rape kit for examination and obtaining legal evidence, keep it within your possession until it is sealed closed. This establishes the legal chain of evidence.

11. Have sexually assaulted patient undress on a clean white sheet and collect any loose foreign articles from the sheet. Place these articles in an envelope provided in rape kit. Label envelope with patient's name, date, and address. Initial, date, and include physician's name.

12. Obtain scrapings from finger nails. Place scrapings in an envelope provided in rape kit. Label envelope as described in procedure number eleven.

13. Obtain a blood sample (for comparison with semen type) with blood tube provided in rape kit. Label appropriately. Additionally, obtain a blood sample for VDRL testing and send to appropriate hospital laboratory or testing facility.

14. Place any soiled or stained articles of clothing in a brown paper bag. Label appropriately; include with rape kit evidence.

15. Comb pubic hair with comb provided in rape kit. Place comb and combings in envelope provided in rape kit. Label appropriately.

16. Cut a small amount of pubic hair with scissors provided in rape kit. Label appropriately.

17. Assist physician with the sexual assault examination:
    a) Remain with patient during the physician's history and physical
    b) Assist physician with the gynecologic examination and collection of evidence. Evidence to be collected is vaginal swab, vaginal smear, and vaginal washings.
    c) Place vaginal smear and vaginal swab in appropriate containers provided in rape kit. Label appropriately.
    d) Assist physician with obtaining gonorrhea culture. Label

appropriately and send to appropriate laboratory or Board of Health.

e) Set aside microscopic slide, with cover slip applied for examination of mobile sperm, for physician

f) Assist physician with rectal examination and collection of evidence (if indicated) of anal smear, anal swab, gonorrhea culture, and microscopic specimen for examination for mobile sperm. Utilize the same procedure and labeling procedure as with vaginal specimens.

g) Assist physician with the oral examination and collection of evidence if indicated. Utilize the same procedure and labeling procedure as with the vaginal specimens.

Follow-Up

1. Administer prescribed medication for prevention of venereal disease, pregnancy, and tetanus
2. Assist with providing treatment for any associated injuries
3. Provide instructions for follow-up appointments and prescriptions
4. Assure patient has adequate physical and psychological support available

Documentation

Patient's physical and emotional status on arrival
Complete description of examination
Treatment administered and prescribed
Notification of Rape Victim Advocates
Follow-up appointments

SUGGESTED READING

Braen RG. Sexual assault. In: Rosen P, Baker FJ II, Braen GR, Dailey RH,

Levy RC, eds. Emergency medicine concepts and clinical practice. Saint Louis: CV Mosby, 1983:1230.

Budassi SA, Barber J. Mosby's manual of emergency care. Practices and procedures. Saint Louis: CV Mosby, 1984:561.

Foley TS, Davies MA. Nursing care of rape victims. Saint Louis: CV Mosby, 1983.

32
STERILE VAGINAL PREPARATION

PAMELA Y. DONNELLY
PAULA K. OVENS

Purpose

To decrease the number of resident bacteria so as to create a safe field of operation. This procedure is aseptic only and not sterilizing.

Indications

- Vaginal procedures such as hysterectomy, laparoscopy, dilatation and curettage, and delivery of infant

Contraindications

- None

Potential Complications

- Allergic reaction to antimicrobial agent

Equipment

Sterile preparation basin (1)
Package of 10 sterile 4×4 gauze sponges (1)
Ring forceps (1)
Moisture proof towel (1)
Pair of sterile gloves (1)
Antimicrobial agent (100 ml) (povidone-iodine, chlorhexidene, etc.)

Procedure

1. Have patient empty bladder prior to beginning preparation
2. Place patient in lithotomy position with head slightly elevated and both feet secured in stirrups
3. Open sterile basin and place 4×4 gauze sponges aseptically into basin
4. Pour antimicrobial agent onto sterile 4×4 sponges
5. Aseptically put on sterile gloves
6. Place moisture proof towel under patient's buttocks
7. Remove two soaked 4×4 sponges from basin
8. Scrub each side of perineal area separately
9. Begin scrub by starting with labia and work outward to include suprapubic area and inside of thigh
10. Discard soiled 4×4 sponges
11. Repeat steps 8-10 for other side of perineal area
12. Spread labia apart with fingers of one hand. Cleanse introitus with two 4×4 sponges
13. Prepare vagina next. Fold two 4×4 sponges into a 2×2 square. Squeeze excessive moisture from sponge. Place folded sponge into the ring forceps.
14. Insert your index and middle finger approximately 1 inch into vaginal canal. Gentle downward pressure (posteriorly) widens the vaginal opening.
15. Insert ring forceps with folded sponge 3-4 inches into vaginal canal and wash all surfaces. Exercise caution when scrubbing vagina to avoid traumatizing tissue.
16. Repeat steps 13-15 using remaining sponges

Follow-Up

1. Ensure clean area for intended procedure

Documentation

Type of preparation done

Indication for preparation
Observe for any adverse reaction to antimicrobial agent

SUGGESTED READING

Clark A, Affonso DD. Childbearing: a nursing perspective. Philadelphia: FA Davis, 1976:403.

Jenson MD, Benson RD, Bobak IN. Maternity care: a nurse and the family. Saint Louis: CV Mosby, 1980:339.

King EM, Wieck L, Dyer M. Illustrated manual of nursing techniques. Philadelphia: JB Lippincott, 1977:291.

MUSCULOSKELETAL PROCEDURES

33

CLOSED REDUCTION

JOY A. GORZEMAN

Purpose

To realign a broken bone
To regain correct alignment
To regain function of the involved part

Indication

- Closed fracture
- Dislocation

Contraindications

- Open fractures

Potential Complications

- Nerve, vascular, or tissue damage

Equipment

Sedative, narcotic, or local anesthesia as ordered
Fixation device

Procedure

1. Explain procedure to patient

2. Administer sedative or analgesic as ordered or assist physician with local nerve block. Allow 5-15 minutes for medication to become effective.
3. Monitor vital signs and patient condition before, during, and after procedure. Pay special attention to pulses distal to injury.
4. Assist physician as necessary while she/he performs manipulation and/or applies traction
5. If physician is unable to perform closed reduction, it will be necessary to admit patient for surgery in order to perform procedure under general anesthesia
6. Obtain x-ray film to check for alignment

Follow-Up

1. Assist in immobilization of reduced extremity with a cast, splint, or traction
2. Provide specific instructions on monitoring and care of extremity, if patient is to be discharged

Documentation

Medication administered and amount
Vital signs and patient response. Special emphasis on color, sensation, and movement in distal extremity.
Follow-up treatment and instructions

SUGGESTED READING

Larson CB, Gould M. Orthopedic nursing. 9th ed. Saint Louis: CV Mosby, 1978:169.
Price SA, Wilson LM. Pathophysiology clinical concepts of disease processes. 2nd ed. New York: McGraw-Hill, 1982:711.
Trafton PG. Fractures. In: Trunkey DD, Lewis FR, eds. Current therapy of trauma-2. Toronto: BC Decker, 1986:335.

34

DRESSINGS AND BANDAGES

BARBARA KALO

Purpose

To promote healing of a wound
To absorb secretions from a wound
To protect area from bacteria, trauma
To immobilize or support an area
To prevent hematoma formation
To improve aesthetics
To reduce painful exposure to the air

Indications

- Open wounds
- Burns

Contraindications

- Dry dressings (if the new epithelium on the wound surface shouldn't be destroyed when removing the dressing)

Potential Complications

- Damage to exposed layer of dermis from drying out of a dressing
- Maceration of skin surface beneath the dressing and bacterial growth with use of occlusive dressing
- Bacterial overgrowth if dressing not changed when soiled or saturated with drainage

- Creation of pressure points with wrinkles in the bandage, especially on extremities
- Restricted circulation

Equipment

Sterile dressings appropriate for wound
Bandage material as needed
Sterile and unsterile gloves
Cleansing solution
Tape
Plastic bag for soiled dressings

Procedure

1. Gather equipment
2. Identify patient
3. Explain procedure
4. Wash hands
5. Remove old dressing with unsterile gloves if applicable, place in plastic bag
6. Don sterile gloves
7. Cleanse wound with sterile solution as ordered
8. Cleanse from center of wound to periphery
9. Apply sterile dressing and secure with tape or bandage material (Fig 34-1)
10. Dispose of used and unused material as necessary

Follow-Up

1. Assess for adequate circulation to affected area
2. Gently wipe away dried blood from area around dressing
3. Assess dressing for proper coverage of wound
4. Assess patient's comfort and proper mobility of affected area

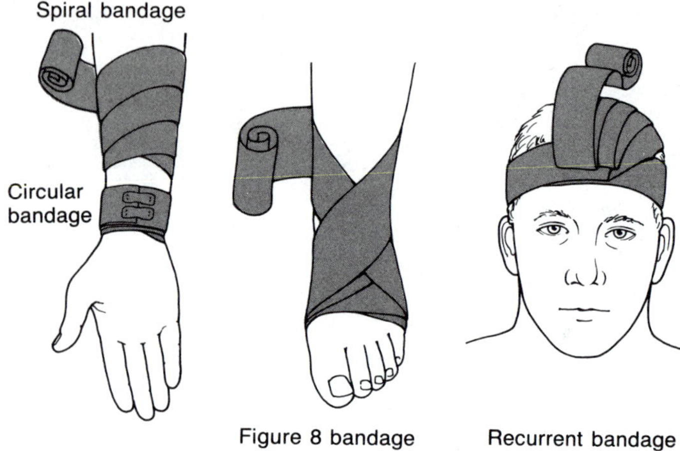

Figure 34–1 Examples of common bandaging techniques.

Documentation

Date and time of procedure

Appearance and size of wound

Estimated amount and character of drainage (note color, type, and odor)

Type of dressing and location

Patient's tolerance to procedure

Instruction to patient and/or family regarding care of dressing or bandage

SUGGESTED READING

Cosgriff JH, Anderson DL. Management of wounds and bites. In: Cosgriff JH, Anderson DL, eds. The practice of emergency nursing. 1st ed. Philadelphia: JB Lippincott, 1975:121.

King E, Wieck L, Dyer M. Illustrated manual of nursing techniques. Bandaging. New York: JB Lippincott, 1977:15

Lewis SM, Collier IC. Medical-surgical nursing: assessment and management of clinical problems. New York: McGraw-Hill, 1983:158.

35

SPLINTING

JOY A. GORZEMAN

Purpose

To prevent damage to nerves, arteries, veins, and soft tissues
To relieve pain

Indications

- Suspected or actual fracture of an extremity

Contraindications

- None

Potential Complications

- If splint is applied too tightly, vascular or nerve damage can occur
- Splint can obscure bleeding, which may lead to shock

Equipment

Depending on the area and type of fracture, there are four common types of splints:
Soft splints such as pillows
Hard splints such as boards
Pneumatic splints (provide support without being held)
Traction splints (provide support and decrease angulation while applying traction)

Procedure

1. Inspect fractured part—check for angulation, shortening, rotation
2. If fracture is open, cover with a sterile dressing
3. Handle fractured part carefully and gently
4. Cut away clothing and/or jewelry, if necessary
5. Check peripheral pulses and assess sensation and motor function
6. Apply splint before patient is moved anywhere
7. Immobilize joint above and below fracture—extend splint well beyond both joints
8. Pad joints with towel or gauze
9. Splint joints in their functional position
10. Do not try to straighten a limb that is severely bent

Follow-Up

1. Check vascular status and temperature of extremity q15min after splinting
2. Check into any complaint of pain or pressure in splinted area
3. Elevate injured extremity after splinting, if not contraindicated by other injuries

Documentation

Type and location of fracture
Type of splint applied
Patient's condition and response to treatment
Vascular status, sensory response, and motor function of affected part

SUGGESTED READING

Brunner LS, Suddarth DS. The Lippincott manual of nursing practice. 3rd ed. Philadelphia: JB Lippincott, 1982:884.

Larson CB, Gould M. Orthopedic nursing. 9th ed. Saint Louis: CV Mosby, 1978:176.

Urosevich PR, ed. Nursing photobook. Dealing with emergencies. Horsham, PA: Intermed Communications, 1982:92.

36

STEINMANN PIN

LISA A. JONES

Purpose

To reduce and immobilize a femur fracture
To decrease muscle spasm
To prevent deformity
To support and maintain alignment

Indications

- Femur fracture

Contraindications

- None

Potential Complications

- Wound tract infection
- Neurovascular compromise
- Skin breakdown

Equipment

Steinmann pin tray
Skin antiseptic solution
4×4 gauze sponges
Weights and ropes
Small needle and syringe

Local anesthetic drug
Pieces of cork or other material to cover pin tips after insertion (2)

Procedure

1. Explain procedure to patient
2. Cleanse area where pin is to be inserted with antiseptic solution
3. Assist physician while area is being anesthetized
4. A small incision is made by physician at site of pin insertion
5. Pin is then inserted with a manual drill device by physician
6. Attach a U-shaped clamp to pin and connect to weights by means of a rope and pulley
7. Apply cork to pin tips to prevent injury to patients or others
8. Apply small dressings at entrance and exit sites of pin

Follow-Up

1. Check for pain, swelling, discoloration, limited motion, numbness, tingling, temperature, position, pulses, and signs of infection
2. Avoid unnecessary movement of weights
3. Ensure proper alignment

Documentation

Patient teaching
Procedure performed and extremity involved
Follow-up assessment
Complications

SUGGESTED READING

Brunner LS, Suddarth DS. The Lippincott manual of nursing practice. Philadelphia: JB Lippincott, 1982:770.

Schwartz S, ed. Fractures and joint injuries. In: Principles of surgery Vol. 2. 4th ed. New York: McGraw-Hill, 1984.

Urosevich PR, ed. Nursing photobook. Dealing with emergencies. Horsham, PA: Intermed Communication, 1980:90.

EYE, EAR, NOSE, AND THROAT PROCEDURES

37

CONTACT LENS REMOVAL

JOY A. GORZEMAN

Purpose

To prevent discomfort or abrasion to the eyes of ill or injured patients who are wearing contact lenses

Indications

- Patients inability to remove own contact lenses

Contraindications

- The possibility of eye injury
- If the colored portion of the eye is not visualized, the lens should only be removed by an eye specialist

Potential Complications

- Corneal abrasions
- Permanent eye damage

Equipment

Containers with labels for storing lenses (2)
Sterile solution for lenses
Eye suction cup, if available

Procedure

Hard Lens (Fig. 37–1)

1. Wash hands. (Hard lenses are most easily removed with suction cup made for that purpose).

   If suction cup is not available:

2. For right eye, stand on right side of patient
3. Place your left thumb lightly on upper eyelid and your right thumb on lower eyelid close to the edge
4. Gently open lids wide, beyond edge of lens
5. Press gently downward with right thumb on the eyeball—the lens should tip
6. Slide eyelids and thumbs together—the lens should come out
7. For left eye, move to left side of patient and repeat steps 2 through 6.
8. DO NOT USE FORCE! If you cannot remove the lens, gently slide it to the sclera and wait for the ophthalmologist.

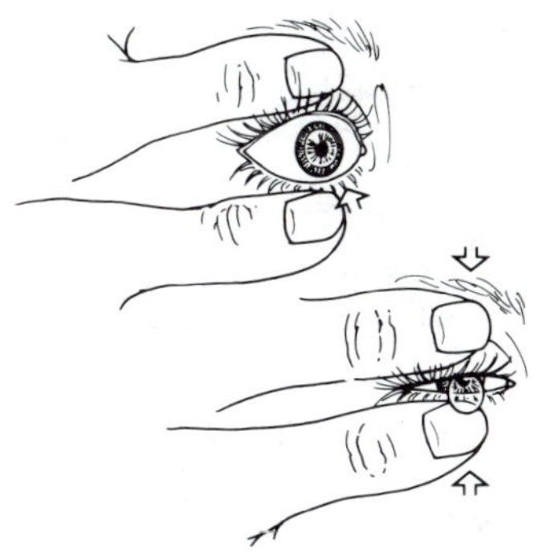

Figure 37–1 Hard contact lens removal (right eye). Open lids wide and press down with right thumb, then slide eyelids together.

Soft Lens (Fig. 37–2)

1. Wash hands
2. Place index finger on rim of lens and slide onto white of the eye
3. Pinch lens between your thumb and index finger and lift it out. Be careful not to rip lens or scratch patient's eyeball with your fingernail.

Follow-Up

1. Place each lens in separate container and label "right" and "left"
2. Soft lenses must be kept moist and should be placed in saline immediately after they are removed
3. Contact lenses are expensive—utmost care should be taken that they are not damaged or lost

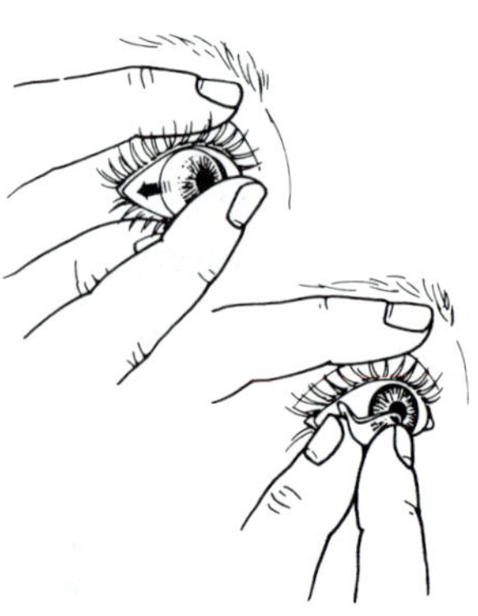

Figure 37–2 Soft contact lens removal (right eye). Slide lens to white of eye and pinch between thumb and index finger.

Documentation

Removal of lenses and where they were placed
If patient is admitted to hospital, note on exterior of chart that patient wears contact lenses

SUGGESTED READING

Brunner LS, Suddarth DS, eds. The Lippincott manual of nursing practice. 3rd ed. Philadelphia: JB Lippincott, 1982:673.
Roth CS, Weaver DT, eds. Pocket manual of emergency medical therapy. 4th ed. Toronto: BC Decker, 1987:104.
Urosevich PR, ed. Nursing photobook. Dealing with emergencies. Horsham, PA: Intermed Communications, 1980:58.

38

EAR IRRIGATION

BARBARA KALO

Purpose

To cleanse and/or remove foreign material from the ear

Indications

- Cerumen impaction
- Foreign body in ear

Contraindications

- Tympanic membrane not intact

Potential Complications

- Ruptured tympanic membrane

Equipment

Irrigation with suction (equipment may vary from a bulb syringe
  to a Water Pik)
Ear forceps
Water at body temperature
Basin to catch fluid
Towel or drape to cover patient's clothing

Procedure

1. Gather equipment
2. Identify patient
3. Explain procedure to patient
4. Wash hands
5. Drape patient
6. Have patient in sitting position
7. Pull auricle up and back
8. Direct flow of solution to top of canal using bulb syringe or Water Pik, if available
9. Dry outside of ear after irrigation

Follow-Up

1. Assess results of irrigation
2. Assess comfort of patient
3. Clean equipment

Documentation

Date and time of procedure
Type and amount of solution
Patient's tolerance to procedure
Character of solution returned
Instructions to patient and/or family as necessary

SUGGESTED READING

Abelson TI, Witt WJ. Otolaryngologic procedures. In: Roberts JR, Hedges JR, eds. Clinical procedures in emergency medicine. 1st ed. Philadelphia: WB Saunders, 1985:916.

Freeman GR. Ear, nose, and throat emergencies. In: Warner CG, ed. Emergency care: assessment and intervention. 2nd ed. Saint Louis: CV Mosby, 1978:349.

Lewis SM, Collier IC. Medical-surgical nursing: assessment and management of clinical problems. New York: McGraw-Hill, 1983:345.

Serio JC. Emergencies involving the ears, nose and throat. In: Cosgriff JH, Anderson DL, eds. The practice of emergency nursing. 1st ed. Philadelphia: JB Lippincott, 1985:423.

39

EYE IRRIGATION

BARBARA KALO

Purpose

To cleanse and/or remove foreign material from the eye

Indications

- Chemical injury to eye
- Foreign body in eye
- Inflammation of eye

Contraindications

- Puncture wound of eye

Potential Complications

- Possible perforating injury to eye if irrigation is not done gently and carefully
- Cross contamination to unaffected eye if infection present
- Abrasion of cornea or conjunctiva

Equipment

Topical anesthetic
Sterile irrigating solution (usually intravenous saline) with tubing
Cotton-tipped applicators
Desmarres retractor (if available)
Gauze pads

Basin
Towel or drape to cover patient's clothing

Procedure

1. Gather equipment
2. Identify patient
3. Explain procedure to patient
4. Wash hands
5. Drape patient
6. Instill topical anesthetic, using Desmarres retractor for lid separation. If not available, eyelid must be held open, using gauze pads.
7. To hold eyelid open, place pressure on bony prominences of cheek and brow, not on eyeball
8. Direct flow of irrigating solution directly over the globe and into the upper and lower fornices, from inner canthus toward outer canthus (Fig. 39-1)
9. Usually 1 liter of fluid is administered rapidly for acid injuries to eyes
10. Usually 2 liters of fluid are indicated for alkaline injuries to eyes

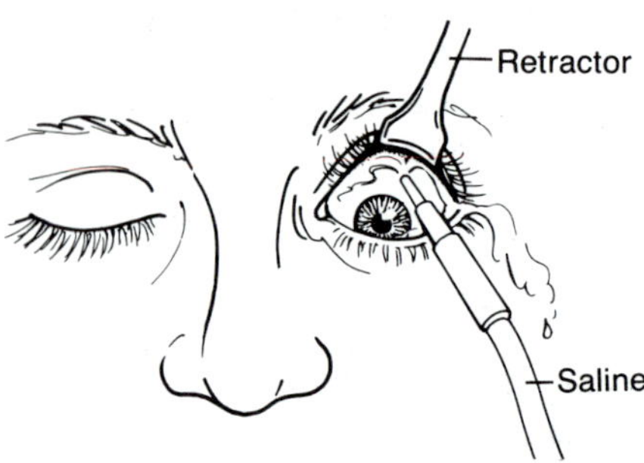

Figure 39-1 Eye irrigation using a Desmarres retractor to separate the lids.

11. Dry outside the eye and surrounding area after irrigation

Follow-Up

1. Check effectiveness of irrigation, measure pH of conjunctival fornices with pH indicator strip
2. The normal pH of the eye is 7.4 and, if measurement is abnormal, continue irrigation
3. If pH is normal, check again after 20 minutes to make sure it remains normal
4. Assess comfort of patient

Documentation

Date and time of procedure
Type and amount of solution
Patient's tolerance to procedure
Character of solution returned, noting any foreign materials
Appearance of eye as to redness, swelling, and pupil reaction
Instructions to patient and/or family as necessary

SUGGESTED READING

Barr DH, Hedges JR. Ophthalmologic procedures. In: Roberts JR, Hedges JR, eds. Clinical procedures in emergency medicine. Philadelphia: WB Saunders 1985:886.

King EM, Wieck L, Dyer M. Irrigation of eye. In: King EM, Wieck L, Dyer M, eds. Illustrated manual of nursing techniques. 1st ed. New York: JB Lippincott, 1977:151.

Schaefer AJ. Care of the patient with ocular injuries. In: Cosgriff JH, Anderson DL, eds. The practice of emergency nursing. 1st ed. Philadelphia: JB Lippincott, 1985:439.

The nursing policy and procedure manual. Dallas: Parkland Memorial Hospital. Policy #6011–29–02.

40

REMOVAL OF FOREIGN BODY FROM THE EAR

NANCY WEINBERG

Purpose

To remove foreign body from the ear

Indications

- Presence of foreign body in ear

Contraindications

- None

Potential Complications

- Lacerations of canal
- Lacerations of tympanic membrane

Equipment

Mineral oil
Local anesthesia (1%):
   Lidocaine, with or without epinephrine (1:100,000)
   ½- to 2-inch # 25 or # 27 gauge needle (1)
   Syringe (3 ml)
Suction catheter (# 3 and # 5)
Speculum
Irrigation syringe with water
Wire loops

Blunt hooks of various sizes
Alligator forceps

Procedure

1. Position patient comfortably
2. Reassure patient
3. Determine nature of foreign body by history and by physician's examination
4. If foreign body is an insect, fill ear canal with mineral oil in order to suffocate insect
5. Assist physician with removal of foreign body from ear. The physician may elect to irrigate, suction, or use mechanical removal.
6. Reassure patient
7. Immobilize patient's head by grasping the patient's head with your hands

Follow-Up

1. Reassure and comfort patient

Documentation

Type of procedure
Success of procedure
Patient's tolerance of procedure

SUGGESTED READING

Abelson TI, Witt WJ. Otolaryngologic procedures. In: Roberts JR, Hedges JR, eds. Clinical procedures in emergency medicine. Philadelphia: WB Saunders, 1985:925.

Birney J, Kulig K, Genta G. Ear, nose, and throat emergencies. In: Kravis TC, Warner CG, eds. Emergency medicine. A comprehensive review. 2nd ed. Rockville, MD: Aspen, 1987:1249.

Budassi SA, Baber J. Mosby's manual of emergency care practices and procedures. 2nd ed. Saint Louis: CV Mosby, 1984:412.

41

REMOVAL OF FOREIGN BODY FROM THE NOSE

NANCY WEINBERG

Purpose

To remove foreign body from the nose

Indications

- Presence of nasal foreign body

Contraindications

- None

Potential Complications

- Aspiration
- Epistaxis
- Trauma to nasal tissue

Equipment

Topical anesthesia and vasoconstriction:
    Topical lidocaine (4%)
    Phenylephrine hydrochloride (0.25%) or
    Cocaine solution (4%) (1 ml)
Suction instrument
Wall or portable suction

Right angle hooks
Alligator forceps or bayonet forceps
Fogarty vascular catheter (# 4)

Procedure

1. Reassure patient
2. Adequately immobilize patient
3. Assist physician during removal of foreign body by assuring immobilization of patient's head

Follow-Up

1. Reassure and comfort patient
2. Control epistaxis (if present)

Documentation

Medications administered
Object removed
Presence and amount of epistaxis
Patient and/or family teaching

SUGGESTED READING

Abelson TI, Witt W. Otolaryngologic procedures. In: Roberts JR, Hedges JR, eds. Clinical procedures in emergency medicine. Philadelphia: WB Saunders, 1985:937.

Birney J, Kulig K, Genta G. Ear, nose and throat emergencies. In: Kravis TC, Warner CG, eds. Emergency medicine. A comprehensive review. 2nd ed. Rockville, MD: Aspen, 1987:1249.

Budassi SA, Barber J. Mosby's manual of emergency care practices and procedures. 2nd ed. Saint Louis: CV Mosby, 1984:413.

42

NASAL PACKING

BARBARA KALO

Purpose

To control nasal bleeding with pressure
To protect cauterized area from drying or trauma
To permit healing of nasal mucosa

Indications

- Anterior and posterior epistaxis

Contraindications

- Usually for a first time bleed

Potential Complications

- Uncontrolled bleeding with poorly placed nasal pack
- Hypoventilation with hypoxia and hypercapnia
- Infection, pain, and dysphagia
- Necrosis of tissue

Equipment

Nasal packing, as ordered
Nasal speculum
Bayonet forceps
Emesis basin
Headlight or head mirror and light

Topical anesthetic and vasoconstrictors
Cotton for topical anesthetic
Towel or drape to cover patient's clothing

Procedure

1. Gather equipment
2. Identify patient
3. Explain procedure to patient
4. Have patient sitting upright
5. Assist physician with procedure:
   a) Anterior packing (Fig. 42–1) is placed in an accordion manner. Each layer is near front of nose.
   b) Posterior packing (Fig. 42–2) consists of either a gauze tampon (placed transorally in nasopharynx, and held in

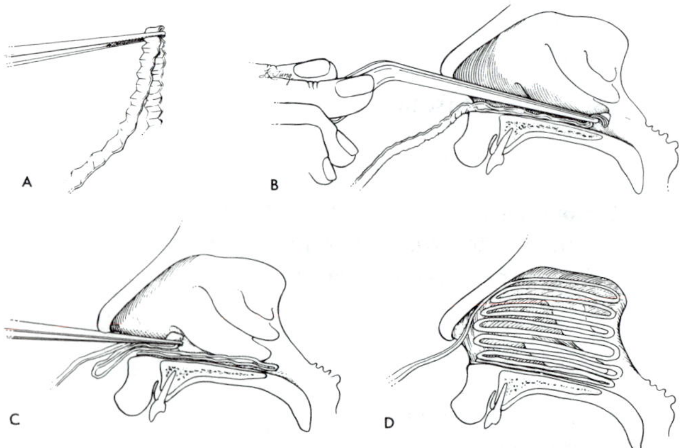

Figure 42–1   Placement of anterior nasal packing. (From Roberts JR, Hedges JR. Clinical procedures in emergency medicine. Philadelphia: WB Saunders, 1985:932.)

place by silk string or umbilical tape) or an inflatable balloon

6. Reassure patient during procedure

Follow-Up

1. Assess for adequate airway
2. Assess for further bleeding after insertion of packing
3. Assess adequate intake by accurate intake and output

Documentation

Date and time of procedure
Type and amount of nasal packing
Patient's tolerance to procedure
Instructions to patient and/or family, as necessary

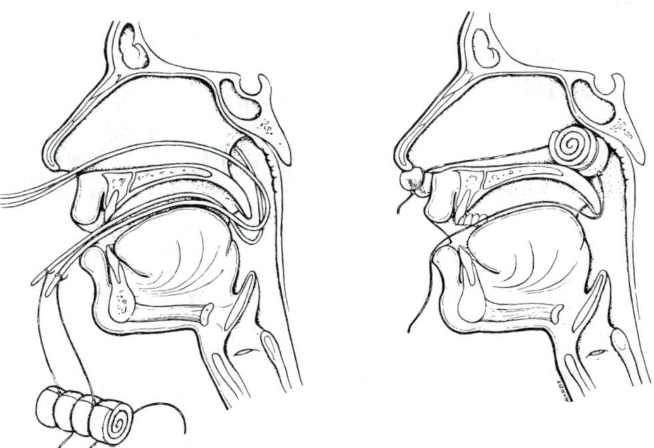

Figure 42–2 Placement of posterior nasal packing. (From Cosgriff JH, Anderson DL. The practice of emergency nursing. Philadelphia: JB Lippincott, 1975:429.)

SUGGESTED READING

Abelson Tl, Witt WJ. Otolaryngologic procedures. In: Roberts JR, Hedges JR, eds. Clinical procedures in emergency medicine. Philadelphia: WB Saunders, 1985:916.

Freeman GR. Ear, nose, and throat emergencies. In: Warner CG, ed. Emergency care: assessment and intervention. 2nd ed. Saint Louis: CV Mosby, 1978:349.

Serio JC. Emergencies involving the ears, nose, and throat. In: Cosgriff JH, Anderson DL, eds. The practice of emergency nursing. Philadelphia: JB Lippincott, 1975:423.

VASCULAR PROCEDURES

43

ARTERIAL BLOOD SAMPLING

KAREN KRENTZ

Purpose

To obtain a blood sample for arterial blood gas (ABG) analysis, which includes the oxygen, carbon dioxide, and bicarbonate content of blood as well as the pH (degree of acidosis or alkalosis)

Indications

- To evaluate and aid in management of hypoxia, acid base balance, and oxygen therapy

Contraindications

- Inadequate collateral circulation to the extremity as evaluated by the Allen's test

Potential Complications

- Hematoma
- Peripheral nerve damage
- Thrombosis
- Arterial spasm
- Impaired circulation to extremity

Equipment

Glass syringe, # 22 or # 23 gauge needle
Heparin (1,000 μg/ml) or a preheparinized syringe
Povidone-iodine pledget
Alcohol pledget
Gauze pad
Cup of ice
Patient identification label
Laboratory requisition
Adhesive bandage strip

Procedure

1. Assemble equipment
2. Heparinize glass syringe by aspirating ½ ml of heparin. Pull back plunger with syringe in a vertical position so as to coat wall of syringe with heparin. Expel air and residual heparin from syringe. A small amount of heparin remains in the hub of the syringe.
3. Identify patient, reassure, and explain procedure
4. Select puncture site—the radial artery is best because it is shallow and there is collateral circulation to the hand. Avoid sites with hematomas, multiple arterial puncture sites, or abnormal skin pathology. Never select a puncture site where distal circulation is compromised. With radial site, the Allen's test should be performed to assess collateral circulation. Ask patient to clench and unclench his fist several times, then occlude the radial and ulnar arteries firmly with your two thumbs. Subsequently, release radial side. One should see a flushing erythema throughout the dorsal surface of the hand, indicating adequate collateral perfusion of the hand.

   Alternate sites include the femoral region, which is easy to palpate but more difficult to maintain hemostasis with such a deep artery. Should there be bleeding after the procedure, there is potential for a serious complication of a large, difficult to detect hematoma. The brachial artery is almost never used because it is the single arterial source to the distal arm.

5. Position wrist so the dorsal surface is exposed. Brace wrist on top of a small towel so that it is firmly positioned in approximately 15 degrees of dorsiflexion. At this time, palpate the artery proximal to the anticipated puncture site with either one or two fingertips. Be certain of where the pulse is, as this is the most important determination to successfully obtain the ABG. Cleanse site with iodine and/or alcohol pledget. Also cleanse the tips of your fingers (Fig. 43–1).

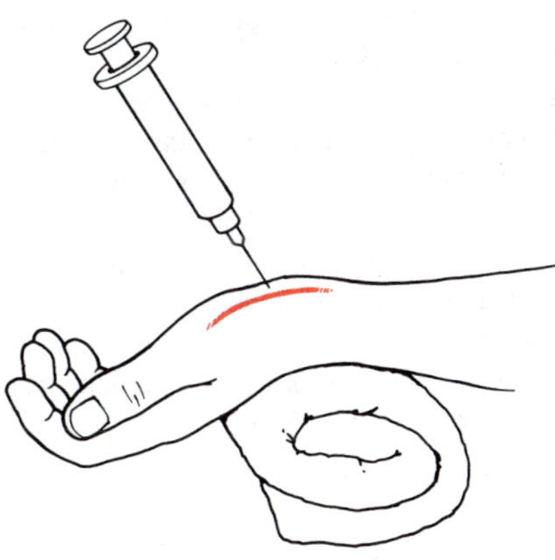

Figure 43–1 Position of wrist for arterial puncture.

6. Position your palpating fingers so that the arterial pulse is easily determined. Then using your other hand, bracing it, puncture the skin at a 30–45 degree angle to the patient's hand. Advance the needle slowly toward the artery until the spontaneous *pulse* of the blood is seen rising and pumping into the syringe. Allow 1–3 ml of blood to enter the syringe. Upon brisk withdrawal of the needle, maintain firm pressure on puncture site for at least 2 minutes.

7. If there is no blood return, withdraw needle slowly until tip is just below surface of the skin and slowly readvance and redirect the needle. (Hint: some nurses prefer to make a swift initial entry with the needle just past where they feel the artery and then slowly withdraw until blood pumps up, in an effort to reduce the pain of the procedure.)

8. Patients who are receiving anticoagulant therapy or who have known clotting disorders must have pressure maintained for at least 10 minutes. Cover puncture site with a sterile adhesive pressure bandage.

9. Expel any air in barrel and replace needle with a syringe cap to prevent air entering syringe and altering measurements

10. Immediately immerse syringe in ice and attach identification label

11. Complete laboratory requisition with a note of any variation of the patient's temperature and percentage of oxygen received, if any

12. Have ABG sample transported to the lab within 15 minutes of its drawing for best results

Follow-Up

1. Observe arterial puncture site for bleeding, hematoma, or distal pallor

2. Assess for blood perfusion in the hand by checking pulse quality, capillary refill, skin color, temperature, and sensation

3. When results of ABGs arrive, analyze them, begin appropriate intervention, and notify physician if indicated

Documentation

Puncture site, results of the Allen's test
Laboratory results, and interventions initiated
Patient's tolerance of procedure
Any additional orders received after notifying appropriate personnel

SUGGESTED READING

American Heart Association. Textbook of advanced cardiac life support. 2nd ed. Dallas: American Heart Association, 1987:181.

Kelly P. Are you ready to perform arterial punctures? Nursing 87 1987; 17(5):39–43.

Miller K. Arterial punctures. In: Millar S, Sampson L, Soukup M, eds. AACN Procedure manual for critical care. 2nd ed. Philadelphia: WB Saunders, 1985:54.

44

ARTERIOGRAM

LISA A. JONES

Purpose

To detect vascular injury

To indicate abnormalities of blood flow due to arterial
obstruction or narrowing

Indications

- Suspected arterial injuries due to trauma
- Suspected vascular insufficiency
- Suspected intracranial arteriovenous malformation or aneurysm

Contraindications

- Allergy to dye used
- Renal insufficiency
- Recent cerebral vascular accident

Potential Complications

- Allergic reaction
- Arterial injury during procedure
- Bleeding
- Renal failure

Equipment

Intravenous catheter and fluid

Procedure

1. Explain procedure to patient

2. Initiate intravenous fluids
3. Consent is obtained by physician and arrangements made with radiologist
4. Patient is transported to radiology department for procedure

Follow-Up

1. On return of patient to Emergency Department, nurse should monitor vital signs q15min × 4, q30min × 4, q1h × 4, then q4h
2. Nurse should also assess distal pulses, for presence and equality, with vital signs
3. Observe site for bleeding and/or hematoma
4. Maintain intravenous fluids
5. Monitor intake and output
6. Instruct patient to remain in low Fowler's position for 6–8 hours after the procedure
7. Prepare patient for surgery if necessary

Documentation

Patient teaching and consent
Time to and from radiology department
Vital signs as per follow-up
Pulses (before and after arteriogram)
Presence or absence of bleeding or hematoma from injection site

SUGGESTED READING

Brunner L, Suddarth D, eds. The Lippincott manual of nursing practice. Philadelphia: JB Lippincott, 1974:318.

Martin-Paredro V. Risk of renal failure after major arteriography. Arch Surg 1983;118:1417–1420.

Tucker S, ed. Patient care standards. Saint Louis: CV Mosby, 1975:112.

45

BLOOD ADMINISTRATION

BARBARA CLARK MIMS

Blood administration involves the transfusion of blood or blood components into the circulation. Appropriate therapy involves the administration of specific blood components to meet specific deficiencies. This procedure addresses only the administration of whole blood and packed red blood cells. (*Appendix B* highlights considerations in the administration of blood components.)

Purpose

To restore circulating blood volume
To improve oxygen-carrying capacity

Indications

- Hemorrhagic shock
- Severe anemia due to blood loss

Contraindications

- None

Potential Complications

- Hypocalcemia
- Hyperkalemia
- Hypothermia
- Microemboli
- Shock
- Viral hepatitis
- Acquired immune deficiency syndrome (AIDS)

- Sepsis
- Circulatory overload
- Renal failure
- Respiratory distress
- Coagulation abnormalities
- Death

Equipment

Venipuncture equipment:
  Tourniquet
  #18 gauge intravenous (IV) catheter
  Iodophor swab
  Iodophor ointment
  Bandage
  Tape
Normal saline (250 ml)
Macrodrop IV administration set with stopcock and extension set
Whole blood or packed red blood cells (as ordered)
Blood recipient set with in-line 170 micron pore filter

Procedure

1. Obtain blood specimen for type and crossmatch. Use tube specified by blood bank, and label carefully with patient's full name, unit number, date, time, and initials of person drawing blood. CAUTION: Carefully check the information on the blood tube with patient's armband. An error during type and crossmatch procedure may result in life-threatening complications.
2. Prepare 250 ml normal saline (NS) by attaching macrodrip administration set, stopcock, and extension set. Prime tubing.
3. Start IV using #18 gauge IV catheter. Begin infusion of normal saline at keep open rate.
4. Obtain unit of blood from blood bank

5. Identify patient by asking him to state his name and then checking his armband
6. Take and record patient's vital signs (blood pressure, pulse, respirations, and temperature) to serve as baseline data
7. Check label on blood bag and requisition form against patient's identification band. Make certain that the following information matches:
   a) Patient's full name
   b) Patient's unit number
   Check to be certain that donor number and ABO and Rh type on blood bag match those on requisition form. Be sure that expiration date on blood bag has not passed. NOTE: This step should be performed by two Registered Nurses or one Registered Nurse and one physician.
8. Carefully insert straight blood recipient set into blood bag. Invert unit and gently squeeze bag to fill entire filter chamber and half of drip chamber with blood.
9. Turn bag upright and prime tubing with blood
10. Check to be sure IV line is patent and that NS is infusing through main IV line. Attach blood tubing to stopcock between IV tubing and extension set. Turn stopcock off to NS and begin to infuse blood slowly (10–15 gtts/min).
11. Observe patient closely for 15 minutes for signs of transfusion reaction (chills, fever, urticaria, itching, back pain, dyspnea, apprehension, hematuria, hypotension)
12. Take and record vital signs 15 minutes after transfusion has begun
13. If no signs of transfusion reaction occur after 15 minutes, set flow rate as prescribed by physician
14. If transfusion reaction is suspected:
    a) Turn off blood infusion. (Do not discard blood or tubing.)
    b) Replace extension set (in order not to infuse blood distal to stopcock). Infuse NS at keep open rate.

c) Notify physician

d) Take and record vital signs

e) Follow hospital protocol for transfusion reaction

15. Take and record vital signs hourly for duration of transfusion. Continue to watch for signs of transfusion reaction.

16. Upon completion of transfusion, flush tubing with NS and remove blood bag and tubing

17. Resume previous IV orders, or discontinue IV as per physician's order

Follow-Up

1. Return empty blood bag to blood bank (if required by institutional policy)

2. Take and record vital signs upon conclusion of transfusion and q4h × 24 hours

3. If additional units of blood are to be hung, check all information specified in #5. In addition, check the ABO and Rh type on blood bag with those on Blood Transfusion Record. If they do not match, notify Blood Bank. One blood filter can be used to administer 2–4 units of blood.

4. Observe for oliguria and jaundice after transfusion therapy

Special Considerations

- Do not administer medications through line while blood is infusing
- Use a blood warmer when blood is transfused at a rapid rate
- Blood must be stored in refrigerator equipped with temperature monitor. Do not place in regular unit refrigerators.
- Do not allow blood to stand longer than 30 minutes at room temperature prior to administering
- Do not allow a unit of blood to hang longer than 4 hours

Documentation

Complete Blood Transfusion Record. Be sure to include donor number, date and time that transfusion was started, and signatures of both nurses who checked the blood.

Vital signs before transfusion was started, 15 minutes after, hourly during the transfusion, and q4h $\times$ 24 hours, following the transfusion

Patient's response to the transfusion. If no signs of transfusion reaction occur, so specify.

Careful intake and output. The volume in each unit of packed red blood cells varies and is specified on the blood bag. Record this volume.

SUGGESTED READING

Brunner LS, Suddarth DS, eds. The Lippincott manual of nursing practice. 3rd ed. Philadelphia: JB Lippincott, 1982:236.

Millar S, Sampson LK, Soukup M. AACN Procedure manual for critical care. Philadelphia: WB Saunders, 1985:409.

Rutman RC, Miller WV. Transfusion therapy principles and procedures. Rockville: Aspen, 1982:40.

Synder EL. Blood transfusion therapy: a physician's handbook. Arlington: American Association of Blood Banks, 1983: 14, 25.

46

CENTRAL VENOUS PRESSURE MONITORING

KAREN KRENTZ

Purpose

To assess the intravascular fluid status of the patient

Indications

- Hypovolemia due to hemorrhage, dehydration

Contraindications

- None

Potential Complications

- Pneumothorax
- Air or catheter tip embolus
- Fluid overload
- Sepsis
- Infection at insertion site
- Pulmonary embolus
- Dysrhythmias

Equipment

Patent central venous line with connected intravenous (IV) setup
Three-way stopcock
Manometer

Procedure

1. Assemble equipment and verify patency of central line
2. Explain procedure to patient
3. Place patient in supine position. If patient cannot tolerate lying flat, place head of bed as low as possible, and mark position of the bed for future central venous pressure (CVP) readings.
4. Locate and mark patient's *zero point* at the level of the right atrium, which is the fourth intercostal space at midclavicular line. The level of the patients head and the zero point must remain constant for readings to be reliable (Fig. 46–1).
5. Using sterile technique, attach CVP manometer to the three-way stopcock so that IV fluid goes into manometer. The port to the patient is closed. The manometer should be filled to approximately 10 mm Hg above the expected reading. (Normal CVP range is 3–12 mm Hg.)

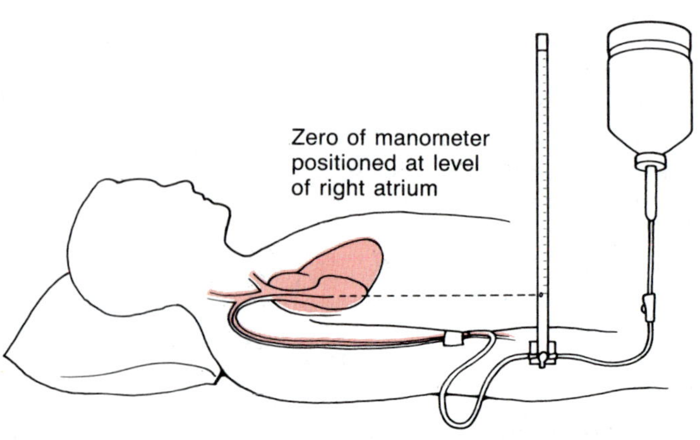

Figure 46–1 Monitoring central venous pressure.

6. To determine CVP measurement, turn stopcock so fluid in manometer runs into patient (the port to the IV fluid is now closed). The fluid in the manometer drops until its equilibrium levels with patient's right atrial pressure. At this point, fluid level fluctuates with patient's respirations because of changes in intrathoracic pressure. The CVP reading is made when patient exhales (the point of lowest intrathoracic pressure).
7. After making the reading, close port to manometer, which opens the IV fluid to the patient

Follow-Up

1. Resume IV drip rate as ordered following the procedure
2. Serially measure CVP (for more consistency)
3. Compare patient's clinical picture to CVP readings, because a number of factors may alter CVP readings. Simultaneous correlation with vital signs, urine output, level of consciousness, and hematocrit should be assessed when evaluating CVP readings.

Documentations

Time of procedure
Results
Resumption of IV flow rate

SUGGESTED READING

Donahue A. Central venous pressure measurement. In: Roberts JR, Hedges JR, eds. Clinical procedures in emergency medicine. Philadelphia: WB Saunders, 1985:332.

Johnson K. Central venous pressure. In: Millar S, Sampson L, Soukup M, eds. AACN Procedure manual for critical care. 2nd ed. Philadelphia: WB Saunders, 1985:81.

Roderick B. How to manage CVP lines. RN 1985; August: 22–25.

47

HEMATOCRIT DETERMINATION

LAURA LUECKE

Purpose

To provide a quick determination of the volume of
packed erythrocytes per deciliter of blood

Indications

- Diagnosis of anemia, polycythemia, oxygen-carrying capacity

Contraindications

- None

Potential Complications

- Altered skin integrity due to punctures
- Incorrect readings

Equipment

Capillary tubes containing anticoagulant
Centrifuge
Microhematocrit reader
Clay-like sealing compound

Procedure

1. Explain procedure to patient

2. Select warm, nonedematous puncture site
3. Clean site with antiseptic and let dry
4. Perform puncture that allows free flow of blood
5. Wipe away first two drops of blood
6. Allow blood to fill at least two capillary tubes to 6–6.5 cm of the 7.5 cm length. Do not overfill.
7. Plug dry end with clay sealing compound
8. Place capillary tubes in centrifuge with clay sealed end at outer edge of centrifuge. Tubes should be placed in a symmetrical pattern in centrifuge.
9. Screw cover on securely, but not so tightly as to break capillary tubes
10. Spin for 3 minutes at high speed (10,000–15,000 G)
11. To read, place capillary tube in groove of plastic indicator on microhematocrit reader so that the bottom of the red cells lines up with the black line on the plastic indicator. Rotate bottom plate so that the 100% line is directly beneath the red line on the plastic indicator, then hold bottom plate in this position. Rotate top plate so that the spiral line intersects the capillary tube at the plasma-air interface. Rotate both discs together until the spiral line intersects the capillary tube at the red cell-white cell interface. Red cell volume in percent is read from point on scale directly beneath the red line of the plastic indicator.

Follow-Up

1. Assess results. When results seem parodoxical, (e.g., low reading after a transfusion) assess patient's volume status.
2. Evaluate for potential sources of error:
   a) Sampling:
      (1) Prolonged tourniquet use causing hemoconcentration
      (2) Hemolysis due to trauma from a fine bore needle
      (3) Inadequate skin puncture

b) Spinning at inadequate speed and duration

c) Inadequate filling or sealing of capillary tube

d) Improper reading

e) Improper interpretation—A change in blood volume may affect hematocrit. The hematocrit may be unreliable immediately after blood loss or blood transfusion. The body may take up to 24 hours to equilibrate.

3. Assess skin integrity. Alternate sites for serial hematocrit punctures.

Documentation

Record results, indicating that the microhematocrit method was used

SUGGESTED READING

Henry JB. Clinical diagnosis and management by laboratory methods. 16th ed. Philadelphia: WB Saunders, 1979:115.

Miale JB. Laboratory medicine: hematology. 6th ed. Saint Louis: CV Mosby, 1982: 360, 383.

Wintrobe MM. Clinical hematology. 8th ed. Philadelphia: Lea & Febiger, 1981:10.

48

INTRAVENOUS CATHETER INSERTION

BARBARA KALO

Purpose

To establish venous access

Indications

- Need for replacement and maintenance of body fluids
- To deliver nutrients and drugs

Contraindications

- Extremity with a shunt or recent surgery

Potential Complications

- Intravenous infiltration
- Air embolus
- Phlebitis
- Hematoma
- Nerve injury
- Local or systemic infection
- Tissue sloughing

Equipment

Intravenous solution as ordered by physician

Intravenous tubing
#18 gauge needle (angiocath)
Tape
Dressing for intravenous site
Alcohol swabs
Labels for intravenous solution
Covered armboard
Intravenous pole

Procedure

1. Gather equipment
2. Identify patient
3. Explain procedure to patient
4. Connect intravenous tubing to intravenous solution
5. Prime tubing by allowing solution to flow through tubing, replacing air
6. Drip chamber should be half full
7. Label intravenous tubing with patient's name, room number, name of intravenous solution, drip rate, name and amount of medication if added, date, time, and nurse's initials
8. Wash hands
9. Select appropriate vein
10. Distend vein:
    a) Have patient open and close fist several times and maintain a closed fist
    b) Lower extremity below patient's heart level
    c) Apply warm towel to area for about 15 minutes if necessary
    d) Slapping the site gently may increase vein prominence
    e) Place tourniquet about 4 inches above level of insertion site
11. Cleanse skin thoroughly with alcohol swab in a circular motion, working from center to outside

12. Pierce skin alongside the vein at a 45 degree angle, bevel up. As needle pierces skin, lower angle of the needle until it is almost parallel with the skin.
13. As blood returns into angiocath, thread catheter into vein while removing needle
14. Remove tourniquet and connect intravenous tubing
15. Tape needle in place with sterile dressing over needle site
16. Set drip rate as ordered

Follow-Up

1. Assess site for swelling, redness, tenderness, or pain
2. Assess drip rate

Documentation

Date, time, site of insertion
Type of intravenous fluid used
Drip rate
Patient's tolerance to procedure
Accurate record of intake and output
Instructions to patient and/or family as necessary

SUGGESTED READING

Coco CD. Intravenous therapy: a handbook for practice. Saint Louis: CV Mosby, 1980:112.

Sager DP, Bomar SK. Intravenous medications: a guide to preparation, administration and nursing management. Philadelphia: JB Lippincott, 1980:22.

The nursing policy and procedure manual. Dallas: Parkland Memorial Hospital, Policy #6011-18-05(11/87).

49

JUGULAR VEIN CANNULATION

KAREN KRENTZ

Purpose

To provide large bore intravenous (IV) access

Indications

- Lack of peripheral IV access
- Need to infuse special medications (i.e., total parenteral nutrition, chemotherapeutics, or multiple simultaneous drug therapies)
- Central venous pressure (CVP) monitoring
- Need for venous access in arrest situations

Contraindications

- Cervical trauma with swelling or anatomic distortion
- Carotid artery disease
- Anatomy of the patient's neck (extremes of weight, short neck)

Complications

- Pneumothorax
- Sepsis (generalized, local cellulitis)
- Hematoma at the neck
- Catheter embolus
- Air embolus
- Dysrhythmias

- Carotid artery puncture
- Fluid overload

Equipment

Central line insertion kit
Intravenous tubing
Intravenous fluid
Appropriately sized intravenous catheter
2–0 silk suture
Xylocaine (1%)
Stopcock
Manometer, if CVP readings ordered

Procedure

1. Assemble equipment
2. Explain procedure and reassure patient
3. Place patient in Trendelenburg position to prevent air embolization and to distend vein. Turn patient's head away from side of intended insertion (Fig. 49–1). Severe rotation makes the internal jugular vein impossible to cannulate without first transversing the carotid artery.
4. Prepare site with iodine solution and drape with sterile towels. The person performing the procedure should wear surgical gloves and a surgical mask.
5. The insertion site may be infiltrated with 1% Xylocaine
6. The jugular vein is cannulated by gently advancing a needle while aspirating for blood with a syringe. A plastic catheter is threaded through the needle and the needle removed. A guide wire (*J-Wire*) may then be advanced through the catheter to allow subsequent placement of a larger or multiple bore catheter.
7. When catheter is in place, attach the primed IV tubing to the

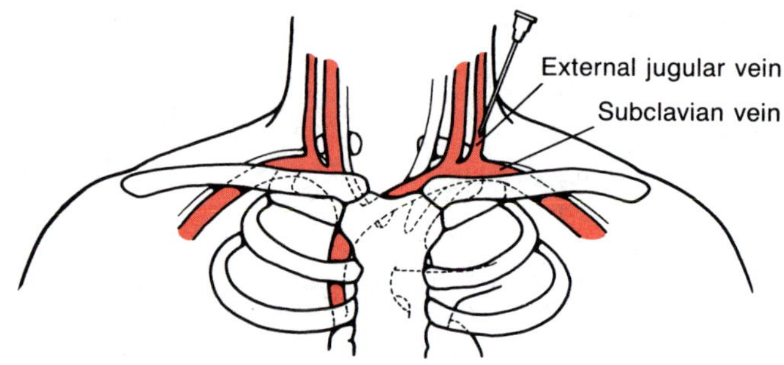

Figure 49–1   Jugular vein cannulation.

hub with the IV flow rate wide open and lower the IV fluid bag below the level of the patient. A prompt venous blood return is observed with successful cannulation.
8. Auscultate for bilateral breath sounds
9. Slow the infusion to a keep open rate until placement of catheter is verified by a stat portable chest x-ray film
10. The catheter is securely sutured to the skin and a topical antimicrobial applied to the site. A sterile occlusive dressing is then applied.

Follow-Up

1. Make sure position of central line has been verified by x-ray film prior to hanging any medications or blood or rapid infusion of fluid
2. Monitor carefully amount of fluid infused and observe for signs of congestive heart failure (because of the capability of infusing large amounts of fluid at a rapid rate, the patient is at risk for volume overload)
3. Monitor closely for patency and constant flow rate. Jugular

lines have a tendency towards kinking because of their position in the neck.

4. Maintain a sterile occlusive dressing to the catheter site for prevention of infection
5. Monitor breath sounds frequently (a pneumothorax may take up to 4 hours to develop)

Documentation

Date and time of procedure
Name of physician
Site of insertion
Type of fluid infusing to each lumen
Verification of blood return to each lumen
Chest x-ray film ordered, completed, and results verified

SUGGESTED READING

American Heart Association. Textbook of advanced cardiac life support. 2nd ed. Dallas: American Heart Association, 1987:141.

Brinkman AJ, Costley DO. Internal jugular venipuncture. JAMA 1973;223:182–183.

Wyte SR, Barker WJ. Central venous catheterization: internal jugular approach and alternatives. In: Roberts JR, Hedges JR, eds. Clinical procedures in emergency medicine. Philadelphia: WB Saunders, 1985:321.

50

SUBCLAVIAN VEIN CANNULATION

KAREN KRENTZ

Purpose

To provide large bore intravenous (IV) access for obtaining central venous pressure (CVP) measurements, instilling special medications (i.e., chemotherapeutics and hyperalimentation), or if there is lack of peripheral IV access

Indications

- Limited venous access
- Dehydration
- Malignancies
- Circulatory collapse

Contraindications

- Pneumothorax
- Bleeding disorders
- Combative patients
- Extremes of weight
- Suspected subclavian vessel injury
- Suspected superior vena cava injury

Potential Complications

- Pneumothorax
- Air or catheter tip embolus

- Fluid overload
- Sepsis
- Infection at insertion site
- Pulmonary embolus
- Dysrhythmias

Equipment

Central line insertion kit
Appropriate central venous catheter
IV fluid
IV tubing
Stopcock
Extension set
Sterile drapes
Towel roll
2–0 silk suture
Xylocaine (1%)
Iodine solution
Crash cart with chest tube

Procedure

1. Assemble equipment. Connect and prime the IV tubing, stopcock, and extension set.
2. Explain procedure to patient
3. With patient in Trendelenburg position, place a towel roll vertically between the patient's scapulas. Turn the head approximately 30 degrees away from the side of intended insertion, usually on the right (Fig. 50–1). This distends the subclavian vein and decreases the risk of air embolization.
4. Prepare the site (sterilely) with an iodine solution and drape with sterile towels. If patient has a thick growth of chest hair, this should be clipped rather than shaved during skin prepa-

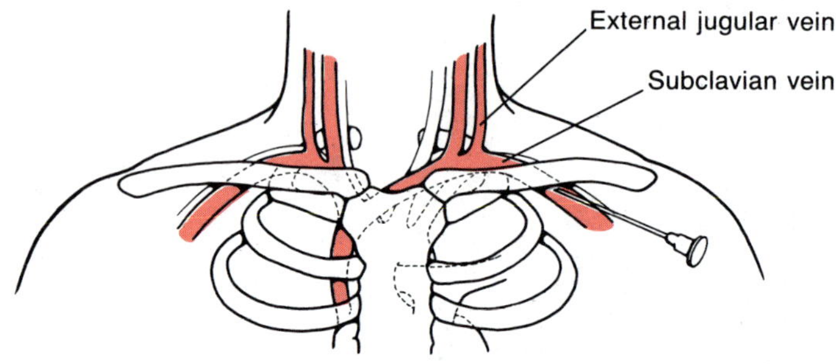

Figure 50–1 Subclavian vein cannulation.

    ration. Large breasts may be taped down away from the field. The person performing the procedure wears gloves and preferably a surgical mask.

5. The insertion site may be infiltrated with 1% Xylocaine for anesthesia

6. The subclavian vein is cannulated by gently advancing a needle while aspirating for blood with a syringe. A plastic cannula is threaded through the needle and the needle removed. A guide wire (*J-wire*) may be advanced through the catheter to allow subsequent placement of a larger or multiple bore catheter.

7. When catheter is in place, attach primed IV tubing to the hub. With IV flow rate wide open, lower the IV bag below the level of the patient. With successful cannulation, a prompt venous blood return is observed.

8. Auscultate chest for breath sounds, bilaterally (i.e., that there is no decrease in breath sounds compatible with pneumothorax).

9. Slow IV fluid to a keep open rate until placement of the central line is verified with a stat chest x-ray film

10. The catheter is securely sutured to the skin and topical antimicrobial applied to the site. A sterile occlusive dressing is then applied.
11. Once line placement is verified by chest x-ray film, proceed with ordered drugs, fluids, and CVP measurements

Follow-Up

1. Frequently assess breath sounds and clinical status for up to 4 hours. (A common complication of subclavian cannulation is a pneumothorax. This may develop as late as 4 hours post-insertion.)
2. Observe, carefully, the amount of fluid infused. (Due to the capability of infusing large amounts of fluid at a rapid rate, the patient with a central line is at risk for volume overload.)

Documentation

Date and time of procedure
Name of physician
Site of insertion
Type of fluid infusing
Verification of blood return
Chest x-ray film ordered, completed, and results verified

SUGGESTED READING

Dronen SC. Subclavian venipuncture. In: Roberts JR, Hedges JR. eds. Clinical procedures in emergency medicine. 1st ed. Philadelphia: WB Saunders, 1985:304.

Dresser DK. Central line insertion. In: Millar S, Sampton L, Soukup M, eds. AACN Procedure manual for critical care. 2nd ed. Philadelphia: WB Saunders, 1985:47.

Nursing policy and procedure manual. Dallas: Parkland Memorial Hospital, 1986. Policy # 6011–18–06.

DIAGNOSTIC PROCEDURES

51

DOPPLER ULTRASONOGRAPHY

LAURA LUECKE

Purpose

To assess the character of blood flow through a vessel

Indications

- To obtain blood pressure readings when auscultation is not reliable
- To assess peripheral arterial and venous blood flow

Contraindications

- Avoid using in vicinity of eye because of the risk of damaging delicate optical nerves

Potential Complications

- Altered skin integrity due to excessive pressure, moisture, or friction
- Inaccurate measurement due to:
  - Inadvertently moving probe off the pulse site
  - Obliterating the blood flow with excessive probe pressure
- Equipment malfunction

Equipment

Doppler-ultrasound device, stethoscope, or automatic speaker
amplifier
Ultrasound transmission gel or water-soluble lubricant

Procedure

1. Apply ultrasound transmission gel or water-soluble lubricant
   to clean faceplate of probe
2. Position probe on skin surface over suspected location of vessel or pulse
3. Tilt probe at approximately a 60-degree angle toward axis
   of blood flow
4. Move probe around site of pulse until pulsatile sound is heard.
   Do not use excessive probe pressure.
5. Mark point at which pulse is heard
6. Obtain blood pressure if desired:
   a) Substitute ultrasound device for stethoscope
   b) Inflate cuff until arterial sound disappears; release cuff
      pressure slowly while checking for auscultatory sound in-
      dicating systolic blood pressure. A diastolic pressure is
      not obtainable with most Doppler devices.

Follow-Up

1. Clean ultrasound probe as directed by the manufacturer
2. Assess skin integrity
3. Record results

Documentation

That ultrasound device was used
Measurements obtained
Changes in measurements

SUGGESTED READING

Durbin N. The application of Doppler techniques in critical care. Focus on Critical Care 1983; 10:44–46.

Kenner CV, Guzzetta CE, Dossey DM. Critical care nursing: body, mind, spirit. 2nd ed. Boston: Little, Brown, 1985:100.

Millar S, Sampson LK, Soukup M. AACN Procedure manual for critical care. 1st ed. Philadelphia: WB Saunders, 1985:182.

52

LEGAL BLOOD ALCOHOL DETERMINATION

LISA A. JONES

Purpose

To obtain blood specimen, for legal purposes, to determine alcohol and/or drug content

Indications

- Written request by a Peace Officer for a blood specimen to be taken for legal purposes (according to the laws of that county)

Contraindications

- Any procedure done without the consent of the patient is technically a battery. Some state statutes grant immunity from civil liability for obtaining blood alcohol levels when a written request is obtained from the officer. The nurse must act on the advice of the hospital attorney, according to his interpretation of the statutes of that state concerning immunity from civil liability. The nurse must also act under the supervision of a licensed physician.

Potential Complications

- None

Equipment

Syringe and needle (or vacutainer needle and holder) and blood specimen tubes

Betadine swab and gauze

Legal forms—request, permit, etc.

Specimen request

Record of patient's signature to consent versus refusal to consent—includes: date, time, officer's name, nurse's name, doctor's name, city and county, and cleansing agent used

Tourniquet

Procedure

1. Skin is prepared with Betadine swab (alcohol swabs should not be used as they might affect laboratory results)
2. Explain to patient that this specimen will be used for legal purposes and obtain written consent
3. Obtain blood in specified tubes
4. Apply gauze to site
5. Label tube with patient's name, age, sex, race, date, and time specimen obtained
6. Label request same as #5 to include type of skin preparation used
7. Attach request tubes and give tubes directly to Peace Officer to protect chain of evidence. These must be taken to the County Toxicology facility.

Follow-Up

1. Observe site for presence of hematoma or bleeding

Documentation

Police department and officer's name who requested procedure

Forms provided by Peace Officers

Patients response to procedure
Betadine preparation used
Date and time specimens obtained
Description of patient's behavior

SUGGESTED READING

DuGas B, ed. Introduction to patient care. 3rd ed. Philadelphia: WB Saunders, 1977:906.

May H, ed. Emergency medicine. 1st ed. New York: John Wiley & Sons, 1984:891.

Miller M, ed. The nurse manager in the emergency department. Saint Louis: CV Mosby, 1983:285.

53

OBTAINING BLOOD SPECIMENS WITH VENIPUNCTURE

CARLA CALLOWAY

Purpose

To obtain blood specimens for laboratory analysis and determination

Indications

- To obtain blood specimens for laboratory analysis and determination

Contraindications

- None

Potential Complications

- Bruising or formation of a hematoma
- Infection
- Nerve injury

Equipment

Vacutainer needle and holder or syringe (size appropriate for amount of blood needed)

Needle (no smaller than #20 gauge)

Vacutainer tubes (type and number determined by tests ordered)

Tourniquet
Povidone-iodine swabs or 70% alcohol swabs
Dry sterile sponges or gauze

Procedure

Vacutainer Method:

1. Gather equipment
2. Wash hands
3. Identify patient, identify self to patient, and explain procedure
4. Apply tourniquet 3–4 inches above puncture site. Do not obtain blood from an area above an intravenous insertion site. (This may cause a distortion in laboratory results because of dilution of blood or electrolytes and/or additives in the intravenous solution.)
5. Palpate for vein. Use povidone-iodine or 70% alcohol swabs to prepare site from which blood is to be collected. (This reduces the number of microorganisms on the skin.) Use povidone-iodine or 70% alcohol swabs to prepare fingertips of person collecting the specimen. (This is to prevent contamination of site while palpating the vein.) Allow skin to dry.
6. Secure needle into holder
7. Insert tube into holder without puncturing tube
8. Apply light tension to skin distal to puncture site with thumb. While continuing to palpate vein with fingers, insert needle, bevel up, at a 30-40 degree angle.
9. Puncture blood tube in holder and stabilize holder
10. Fill each tube until necessary amount of blood is obtained. Carefully remove each tube and replace with another until all tubes are filled with necessary amount of blood. (Fill anticoagulant tubes first, ending with clotted specimens. Anticoagulant tubes must be filled to exhaustion of vacuum to ensure proper ratio of anticoagulant to blood. Immediately

after filling, invert tubes with blood and anticoagulants several times to mix.)

11. Remove last tube from holder
12. Release tourniquet
13. Withdraw needle while applying pressure to venipuncture site with gauze
14. Apply pressure to site until bleeding has stopped

Syringe Method:

1. Secure needle onto syringe
2. Fully depress syringe plunger
3. Apply slight tension to skin distal to puncture site with thumb. While continuing to palpate vein with fingers, insert needle, bevel up, at a 30-40 degree angle.
4. Gently pull back on plunger with one hand to withdraw necessary amount of blood. Use other hand to stabilize syringe barrel. Use minimal amount of suction to prevent hemolysis of blood and collapse of vein.
5. When necessary amount of blood has been obtained, release tourniquet
6. Withdraw needle while applying pressure to venipuncture site with gauze
7. Apply pressure to site until bleeding has stopped
8. Fill all tubes with necessary amount of blood. (Fill anticoagulant tubes first, ending with clotted specimens. Anticoagulant tubes must be filled to exhaustion of vacuum to ensure proper ratio of anticoagulant to blood. Immediately after filling, invert tubes with blood and anticoagulants several times to mix.)

Follow-Up

1. All blood tubes should be labeled with the following information:
   a) Patient's full name

    b) Date and time blood was collected

    c) Initials of person who collected blood

    d) Any other necessary identification (i.e., identification numbers, patient location, doctor's name, etc.)

    e) Any precautions or other pertinent information that laboratory personnel should be aware of (i.e., infectious diseases transmitted in the blood)

2. Attach appropriate labels and requisitions to all blood specimens and see that specimen is delivered to proper laboratory
3. Monitor puncture site for signs of continued bleeding
4. Properly dispose of needle and syringe in appropriate receptacles
5. Wash hands

Documentation

Time blood specimens were collected

Venipuncture site and any excessive measures needed to stop bleeding

Types of test to be done on collected blood

SUGGESTED READING

Brunner LS, Suddarth DS, eds. The Lippincott manual of nursing practice. 3rd ed. Philadelphia: JB Lippincott, 1982:94, 98, 234.

French RM. Guide to diagnostic procedures. New York: McGraw-Hill, 1975:58.

Hamilton HK, ed. Diagnostics: nurse's reference library series. Springhouse: Intermed Communications, 1981: XXVI.

Smith D. Diagnostic procedures: the patient and the health care team. New York: John Wiley & Sons, 1983:23.

54

THROAT CULTURE

BARBARA KALO

Purpose

To detect the presence of pathogens and the organism's sensitivity to specific antibiotic agents

Indications

- Inflamed, congested, painful throat

Contraindications

- Laryngeal spasms

Potential Complications

- None

Equipment

Sterile culture tube with media
Sterile swab
Tongue depressor

Procedure

1. Gather equipment
2. Identify patient
3. Explain procedure to patient

4. Wash hands
5. Hold down tongue with depressor
6. With sterile swab, wipe posterior pharyngeal wall as well as tonsillar area
7. Replace swab in media culture tube
8. Affix proper label to collection tube
9. Send specimen to laboratory

Follow-Up

1. Assess patient for adequate airway

Documentation

Date and time of procedure
Appearance of throat
Exudate noted
Patient's tolerance of procedure
Disposition of specimen
Instructions to patient and/or family as necessary

SUGGESTED READING

Abelson TI, Witt WJ. Otolaryngologic procedures. In: Roberts JR, Hedges JR, eds. Clinical procedures in emergency medicine. 1st ed. Philadelphia: WB Saunders, 1985:916.

Suddarth DS, Brunner LS, eds. The Lippincott manual of nursing practice. 2nd ed. New York: JB Lippincott, 1978:15.

The nursing policy and procedure manual. Dallas: Parkland Memorial Hospital. Policy #6011–26–09 (11/87).

55

WOUND CULTURE

BARBARA KALO

Purpose

To detect the presence of pathogens and the organism's sensitivity to specific antibiotic agents

Indications

- Infection at wound site

Contraindications

- None

Potential Complications

- Reinfection of another area if sterile technique is broken

Equipment

Sterile culture tube with media and swab
Sterile and nonsterile gloves
Sterile dressing appropriate for wound
Tape
Plastic bag for soiled dressing

Procedure

1. Gather equipment

2. Identify patient
3. Explain procedure to patient
4. Wash hands
5. If applicable, don nonsterile gloves, remove old dressing, and discard in plastic bag
6. With sterile swab, wipe wound in area of exudate if possible
7. Replace swab in media culture tube
8. Affix proper label to collection tube
9. Send specimen to laboratory
10. Wash hands
11. Don sterile gloves
12. Apply sterile dressing and secure with tape
13. Dispose of used and unused material as necessary

Follow-Up

1. Assess patient's comfort
2. Assess proper placement of dressing

Documentation

Date and time of procedure
Appearance and size of wound
Note color, type, and odor of drainage
Disposition of specimen
Type of dressing and location, if applicable
Patient's tolerance to procedure
Instruction to patient and/or family

SUGGESTED READING

King EM, Wieck L, Dyer M. Illustrated manual of nursing techniques. 1st ed. New York: JB Lippincott, 1977:127.

Pfaff SJ, Wound management: clean wounds. In: Millar S, Sampson LK, Soukup SM, eds. AACN Procedure manual for critical care. 2nd ed. Philadelphia: WB Saunders, 1985:433.

The nursing policy and procedure manual. Dallas: Parkland Memorial Hospital. Policy #6011–26–09 (11/87).

OTHER PROCEDURES

56

BURN CARE

LISA MORRA-MARTIN

Purpose

To determine extent of burn
To provide initial supportive or resuscitative care to the burn patient

Indications

- Chemical, electrical, or thermal burns

Contraindications

- None

Complications

- As noted in procedure

Procedure

Life Saving Measures:
1. Upon arrival, perform a brief assessment of victim's airway, noting respiratory rate and character to ensure that airway is not obstructed
2. Stop burning process by removing all clothing and checking for smouldering fabric

3. Cover patient with clean dry sheet
4. Avoid cold and ice
5. Institute immediate lavage of chemical burns using either specific neutralizing agents, saline, or tap water as ordered

Patient History and Nursing Assessment:
1. Obtain a history of accident from patient, family, or rescue squad
2. Determine exact time of injury and circumstances surrounding injury
3. Obtain a brief medical history, including any allergies, preexisting medical conditions, and present medications
4. Obtain a complete set of vital signs
5. Perform a systems assessment and evaluate patient for associated injuries
6. Determine patient's height and weight

Evaluation of Airway:
1. Evaluate both upper and lower airway
2. Note presence of facial burns, singed nasal hair, edema of pharynx and/or nasal septum, mucosal redness, presence of carbonaceous sputum
3. Make special notation of early facial swelling, hoarseness, and disorientation. If patient experiences any of the aforementioned signs or symptoms, prepare for intubation and possible ventilatory assistance. (See *Oral Airway Insertion* and *Endotracheal Intubation*)
4. Monitor patient status and obtain serial arterial blood gases
5. Provide oxygen therapy as ordered; observe if patient's vital signs are stable and arterial blood gases acceptable
6. Provide high flow oxygen devices as ordered for those patients suffering from carbon monoxide poisoning

Assessment and Calculation of the Burn Injury:

1. Assess depth of burn (Table 56–1) and estimate and calculate the extent of injury by applying the Rule of Nines (Fig. 56–1).

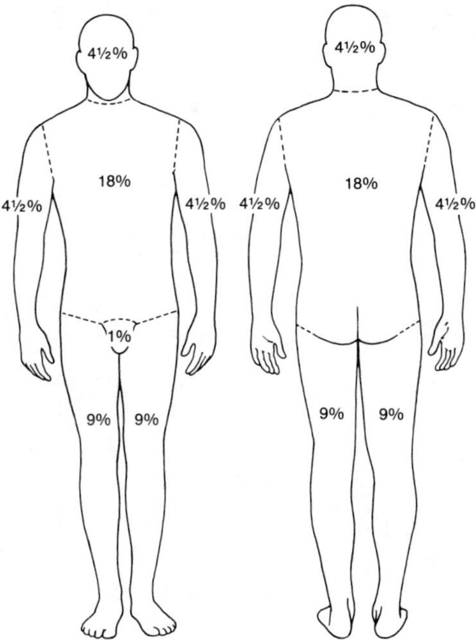

Figure 56–1 Estimating burns using the Rule of Nines. (Adapted from Morra LB. Burns. In: Mancini M. Decision making in emergency nursing. Toronto: BC Decker, 1987:66.)

Table 56-1 Depth of Injury of Burn

Degree	Mechanism of Injury	Appearance	Sensation	Healing
First	Exposure to sunlight or minor flash	Red Dry	Painful	3–5 days without scarring
Second	Limited exposure to hot liquids, objects, flash, flame, or chemical agent	Red to pale ivory Moist, weeping, formation of blisters	Painful	10–20 days with variable amounts of scarring
Third	Prolonged exposure to flame, hot objects, or chemical agents High voltage electrical injury	White, charred red, or cherry red Dry, hard, leathery May see thrombosed veins and deep blisters	Insensitive	Requires grafting

NOTE: The rule does not apply to children. A more accurate assessment of the area involved may be obtained by employing the Lund-Browder chart, which takes into consideration variations in body proportions with age. It is helpful to remember when calculating burns of irregular border that one surface of the patient's hand is equal to approximately 1 % of body surface (Fig. 56–2).

2. The patient should then be triaged and managed according to the following general guidelines:
   MINOR BURNS:
   Can usually be treated as outpatient and include:
   a) Second degree burns of less than 15 % in adults
   b) Second degree burns of less than 10 % in children
   c) Third degree burns of less than 2 %
   MODERATE BURNS:
   Should be admitted and treated in a community or general hospital and include:
   a) Second degree burns of more than 10–30 % in adults
   b) Second degree burns of more than 10–20 % in children
   MAJOR BURNS:
   Should be admitted to a major burn treatment center and include:
   a) Second degree burns exceeding 30 %
   b) Third degree burns exceeding 10 %
   c) Burns involving the face, hands, feet, or perineum
   d) All victims with associated medical conditions such as diabetes, cardiorespiratory disease, inhalation injury, chemical or electrical burns
3. Administer tetanus immunization

AREA	Inf.	1–4	5–9	10–14	15	Adult	Part	Full	Total	Donor Areas
Head	19	17	13	11	9	7				
Neck	2	2	2	2	2	2				
Ant. Trunk	13	13	13	13	13	13				
Post. Trunk	13	13	13	13	13	13				
R. Buttock	2½	2½	2½	2½	2½	2½				
L. Buttock	2½	2½	2½	2½	2½	2½				
Genitalia	1	1	1	1	1	1				
R.U. Arm	4	4	4	4	4	4				
L.U. Arm	4	4	4	4	4	4				
R.L. Arm	3	3	3	3	3	3				
L.L. Arm	3	3	3	3	3	3				
R. Hand	2½	2½	2½	2½	2½	2½				
L. Hand	2½	2½	2½	2½	2½	2½				
R. Thigh	5½	6½	8	8½	9	9½				
L. Thigh	5½	6½	8	8½	9	9½				
R. Leg	5	5	5½	6	6½	7				
L. Leg	5	5	5½	6	6½	7				
R. Foot	3½	3½	3½	3½	3½	3½				
L. Foot	3½	3½	3½	3½	3½	3½				
									TOTAL	

Figure 56–2 Estimating burns using the Lund-Browder chart.

Management of Major Burns:

1. Insert two large bore IV catheters, preferably in upper extremities. Unburned skin sites are desirable. (See *Intravenous Catheter Insertion*.)

2. Draw admission blood work, which should include arterial blood gases, electrolytes, and complete blood count

3. Determine fluid volume of Ringer's lactate solution for resuscitation during the first 24 hours post-injury by the following formula:

4 ml/kg of body weight/percent burn

NOTE: Several investigators have indicated through studies that during the initial 24 hours post-burn, colloid containing fluids are not imperative for resuscitation. It appears that such fluids exert no greater restorative effect on cardiac output nor are such fluids retained within the circulation to a greater extent than an equal volume of colloid-free electrolyte containing fluid such as Ringer's lactate. Therefore to achieve the goal of vital organ function maintenance at minimal cost, a balanced salt solution for fluid replacement is recommended during the first 24 hours post-burn.

4. Administer half the total amount during the first 8 hours from the time of injury

5. Administer the remaining half over the succeeding 16 hours

   EXAMPLE: A 70 kg patient is admitted with a 60 % total body surface area burn.

   The patient would receive a total of 16,800 ml (4 ml × 70 × 60) of Ringer's lactate in the first 24 hours post-burn. In the first 8 hours, 8,400 ml would be delivered. Over the succeeding 16 hours, 8,400 ml would be delivered.

   NOTE: If greater than 50 % total body surface area burn, the patient requires approximately 20 % more than the calculated amount of fluid. Other factors such as delayed resuscitation, inhalation injury, soft tissue injury, escharotomies, and liver disease may also affect fluid resuscitation.

6. Insert a nasogastric tube and evacuate the stomach. (See *Nasogastric Intubation.*)

7. Insert a Foley catheter with a urometer to permit hourly determinations of urine output. (See *Urethral Catheterization.*) NOTE: IV fluid rates should be adjusted as ordered to maintain urine output at 40–70 ml/hr in adults. Victims of electrical injuries characteristically have large amounts of hemochrogens in their urine, which further predisposes these patients to acute renal failure. As a result, if such pigment concentration exists, fluid should be infused at a rate necessary to achieve an hourly urine output of 75–100 ml. If such treatment is unsuccessful, 12.5 g of Mannitol may be administered to each liter of IV fluid, as ordered, until urine output is at a desirable level and the pigment clears.
8. Obtain an electrocardiogram on those patients sustaining an electrical burn. (See *Electrocardiogram: 12 Lead.*)
9. Perform peripheral circulation evaluations, assessing pulses, tactile sensation, numbness, motion, and deep pain, of those patients with circumferential third degree burns of the extremities. Remove all jewelry such as rings and watches.

Follow-Up

1. Monitor ventilatory status frequently in those patients with full thickness burns of the thoracic wall
2. Elevate uncompromised burned extremities and check pulses qlh × 24 hours
3. Elevate compromised burned extremities and prepare for escharotomies
4. Continue to evaluate hourly vital signs, urine output, sensorium, ventilation, and status of fluid administration
5. Continuously monitor patient until transfer to an intensive care unit

Documentation

Initial and ongoing assessment with emphasis on airway and burn
status
Procedures undertaken and patient response

SUGGESTED READING

Baxter CR. Problems and complications of burn shock resuscitation. Surg Clin
North Am 1978; 58 (6):1313–1322.

Fisher SV, Helm PA. Comprehensive rehabilitation of burns. Baltimore: Williams & Wilkins, 1984.

Hunt JL, Sato RM, Baxter CR. Acute electrical burns: current diagnostic and
therapeutic approaches to management. Arch Surg 1980; 115:434–438.

Luterman A, Curreri PW. Emergency treatment of burn injuries. Hosp Med
1980; 16 (1): 66–79.

Moncrief JA. Burns I: assessment. JAMA 1979; 242 (1):72–74.

Moncrief JA. Burns II: initial assessment. JAMA 1979; 242 (2):179–182.

Moore E, Eiseman B, Van Way CW III. Critical decisions in trauma. Saint
Louis: CV Mosby, 1984.

Munster AM. The early management of thermal burns. Surgery 1980; 87:29–40.

Sabiston DC. The textbook of surgery. Philadelphia: WB Saunders, 1986:214.

Salisbury RE, Newman NM, Dingeldein GP Jr. Manual of burn therapeutics.
Boston: Little, Brown, 1983.

Trunkey DD. Inhalation injury. Surg Clin North Am 1978; 58:1133–1140.

57

CARDIOPULMONARY RESUSCITATION

MARY E. MANCINI

Purpose

To provide artificial ventilation and circulation so as to provide oxygen to the brain, heart, and other vital organs until definitive medical treatment can be initiated

Indications

- Cardiopulmonary arrest

Contraindications

- None

Potential Complications

- Aspiration
- Gastric distention
- Laceration of internal organs
- Rib fractures

Equipment

Bag-valve-mask unit
Cardiopulmonary resuscitation record
Supplemental oxygen

Procedure

1. Assess patient for unresponsiveness by gently shaking and calling loudly, "Are you OK?" Caution should be used in shaking any trauma victim.
2. If patient does not respond, assure adequate assistance is available
3. Open airway. Move lower jaw forward, using head-tilt-chin-lift maneuver or the jaw-thrust maneuver. This lifts the tongue away from the back of the throat and prevents obstruction.
4. Determine breathlessness. While maintaining an open airway, place your ear over patient's nose and mouth and observe patient's chest. Look for chest to rise and fall, listen for exhalation and feel for flow of air. If after 3-5 seconds none of the aforementioned are noted, prepare to initiate artificial respiration. A bag-valve-mask unit should be used whenever possible to ventilate the apneic patient. However, if one is not available, mouth-to-mouth rescue breathing should be started.
5. **If bag-valve-mask unit is available:**
    a) The bag-valve-mask unit should be used only by well trained and experienced personnel as it is difficult to maintain an open airway while providing adequate ventilation volume
    b) The head must be maintained in extension with the jaw elevated and the mask held tightly against the patient's face. Therefore, the nurse should be positioned at the head of the stretcher. One hand is used to hold the mask in place and the head in position. The other hand is used to squeeze bag.

    If a bag-valve-mask is not available:
    a) Pinch patient's nose closed using thumb and index finger of the hand placed on the forehead and used to maintain the head-tilt

b) Taking a deep breath, form an airtight seal with your mouth over patient's mouth

6. Deliver two full breaths—each lasting 1½ seconds/breath. Adequate time should be allowed to ensure good chest expansion and decrease likelihood of gastric distention. Supplemental oxygen should be added as soon as possible.

7. Determine pulselessness by locating carotid artery and checking for a pulse. This can be accomplished while maintaining the head-tilt with one hand on the forehead, locating the patient's larynx with two fingers of the other hand, and sliding the fingers into the groove between the trachea and the muscles at the side of the neck. To avoid compressing the artery, press gently for at least 5 seconds. Adequate time should be given to assure if a slow, irregular, or weak pulse would be identified.

8. If pulseless, perform external chest compressions with hands located on the lower half of sternum, arms straight, elbows locked, and shoulders over your hands. Perform compressions at rate of 80–100 per minute.

9. During two person CPR, deliver one breath during a pause after every fifteen chest compressions. Breath should last 1 to 1½ seconds.

10. Assess patient frequently to assure that CPR is generating an artificial pulse

11. After every therapeutic intervention, stop CPR and assess patient to determine if a spontaneous pulse has returned

Follow-Up

1. If not yet done, place patient on monitor, initiate intravenous line and follow vital signs q5–10min until stable

2. Determine cause for cardiac arrest, and assist in stabilizing patient

3. Assess patient for potential complications

4. Provide information and support to family as appropriate

Documentation

Time of initiation and duration of CPR
Patient responses to therapy

SUGGESTED READING

American Heart Association. Standards and guidelines for cardiopulmonary resuscitation and emergency cardiac care. JAMA 1985; 255:2915–2922.

Babbs CF. Practical advances in cardiopulmonary resuscitation. In: Callaham, ML, ed. Current therapy in emergency medicine. Toronto: BC Decker, 1987:38.

Brunner LS, Suddarth DS, eds. The Lippincott manual of nursing practice. 3rd ed. Philadelphia: JB Lippincott, 1982:863.

Niemann JT. Improving systemic perfusion during cardiopulmonary resuscitation. In: Callaham ML, ed. Current therapy in emergency medicine. Toronto: BC Decker, 1987:43.

Roth CS, Weaver DT, eds. Pocket manual of emergency medical therapy. 4th ed. Toronto: BC Decker, 1987:215.

58

INTRAVENOUS MEDICATION ADMINISTRATION

BARBARA KALO

Purpose

To administer medication via intravenous (IV) line for rapid effect

Indications

- To relieve pain quickly
- To begin treatment of infection with antibiotics
- To relieve symptoms of an illness with therapeutic medications
- To induce drowsiness

Contraindications

- Known allergy to medication

Potential Complications

- Incompatibility of medication with IV solution
- Air embolus
- Extravasation
- Toxic reaction or shock if too rapid absorption of a drug

Equipment

Medication as ordered
Individual 50–100 ml bag of dextrose and water or normal saline
    or a volume control set

IV tubing for individual bag
Labels for volume control set or individual bag
Alcohol swabs
#21 gauge needles

Procedure

1. Gather equipment
2. Identify patient
3. Explain procedure to patient
4. Wash hands
5. Fill volume control set with appropriate amount of fluid for dilution of medication
6. Cleanse injection port with alcohol swab, and inject medication into volume control set
7. Connect volume control set to stopcock in main IV line or attach #21 gauge needle to tubing and insert into injection port of IV tubing, after cleansing with alcohol
8. If using individual bag, inject medication after cleansing injection port with alcohol
9. Connect tubing to bag and connect to stopcock in main IV line or attach #21 gauge needle to tubing and insert into injection port of IV tubing, after cleansing with alcohol
10. Thoroughly mix medication in the volume control set or individual bag by turning upside down and shaking
11. Label volume control set or individual bag
12. Regulate drip rate—most IV piggyback medications should be infused in 20–30 minutes
13. To inject medication directly, cleanse injection port with alcohol and inject as rapidly or slowly as directions indicate after assessing a good blood return

Follow-Up

1. Assess IV site for redness, swelling, tenderness, or pain

Documentation

Date and time
Medication
Method of administration
Patient's tolerance to procedure
Instructions to patient and/or family as necessary

SUGGESTED READING

Coco CD. Intravenous therapy: a handbook for practice. 1st ed. Saint Louis: CV Mosby, 1980:55.

Sager DP, Bomar SK. Intravenous medication: a guide to preparation, administration, and nursing management. 1st ed. Philadelphia: JB Lippincott, 1980:110.

The nursing policy and procedure manual. Dallas: Parkland Memorial Hospital. Policy #6011-20-06 (07/87).

59

MANAGING COMBATIVE PATIENTS WITH PHYSICAL RESTRAINTS

JERRY BROCK

Purpose

To immobilize a patient who is unable to control aggressive impulses

To prevent the patient from injuring self or others

To prevent the patient from removing treatment devices

Indications

- When verbal interventions are not successful in preventing the patient from losing control
- When the patient demonstrates:
  - Motor restlessness
  - Accelerated use of profanity
  - Posture indicating a fighting stance
  - Increased pacing
  - Increased delusional and paranoid thinking
  - Threatening hallucinations

Contraindications

- Restraints should not be used for punishment or to immobilize a patient in order to free staff from responsibility of observations

Potential Complications

- Bruises and abrasions
- Restriction of circulation
- Vomiting with aspiration
- Suffocation

Equipment

Soft restraints
Vest restraints
Leather restraints
Full body restraint

Procedure

General Information:

1. Ensure adequate number of personnel are available to accomplish task safely
2. Each member of the team is assigned a specific responsibility during procedure
3. Inform patient that restraints are being applied because he is unable to control behavior and that restraints will be removed as soon as he is able to regain control
4. Administer medications
5. Never fasten restraints to side rails
6. Only apply restraint in a horizontal line and maintain proper body alignment
7. Remove restraints as soon as patient's condition permits

Soft Restraints

1. Place cuff around limbs. Follow directions on package for securing.
2. Assess distal circulation
3. Secure straps to bedframe or chair

4. Tie a bow or knot that can be released quickly

Vest Restraint:

1. Assist patient to sitting position
2. Slip vest over gown
3. Apply vest as outlined on package
4. Do not restrict respirations by wrapping vest too tightly
5. Secure straps, leaving 1–2 inches of slack

Leather Restraints:

1. Place restraints across bed under patient's extremities in position for cuffs to receive wrist and ankles
2. Position wrist and ankles through restraining holder and adjust size
3. Secure to bed frame

Full Body Restraint:

1. Place patient in supine position
2. Cover patient with netting
3. Slip appropriate opening over head and limbs
4. Position wrist and ankles into cuffs and secure

Follow-Up

1. Do not leave patient alone
2. Monitor vital signs
3. Turn patient q2h, and provide full range of motion except during sleep
4. Provide fluids frequently
5. Feed patient if restraints inhibit self feeding
6. Offer bedpan or urinal or take patient to the bathroom q4h or prn
7. Remove one limb at a time, and provide skin care q4h

8. Assess circulation q30min
9. Reassure and comfort patient

Documentation

Behaviors exhibited requiring restraints
Type of restraint used
Patient's response to procedure
Follow-up care

SUGGESTED READING

Beck C, Rawlins R, Williams S. Mental health–psychiatric nursing. Saint Louis: CV Mosby, 1984:1065.
Brunner LS, Suddarth DS, eds. The Lippincott manual of nursing practice. 3rd ed. Philadelphia: JB Lippincott, 1982:976.
Janosik E, Davies J. Psychiatric mental health nursing. Boston: Jones & Bartlett, 1976:415, 621.

60

NITRONOX ADMINISTRATION

LISA A. JONES

Purpose

To provide analgesia for alert patients complaining of moderate
to severe pain

Indications

- Fractures
- Kidney stones
- Burns
- Surgical procedures

Contraindications

- Chest injuries
- Head injuries
- Chronic obstructive pulmonary disease
- Drunkenness
- Pediatrics
- Maxillofacial injuries
- Manic patients
- Patients unable to self-administer Nitronox
- Hypotensive patients
- Hypertension

Potential Complications

- Hypotension
- Hypertension

Equipment

Nitronox tank and mask
50% nitrous oxide and 50% oxygen is considered optimal

Procedure

1. Check both tanks (nitrous and oxygen) prior to use, to ensure both are filled and functioning
2. Inform patient of purpose of Nitronox
3. Instruct patient to administer Nitronox to himself by placing mask tightly against face and breathing slowly and deeply. When adequate sedation is acheived, the patient becomes drowsy and drops the mask from his face preventing over medication.
4. Stay with patient during procedure
5. Monitor vital signs before, during, and after administration

Follow-Up

1. Check vital signs

Documentation

Vital signs before, during, and after administration
Patient response (i.e., pain relieved)
That medication was self-administered for the purpose of analgesia
Complications during procedure

SUGGESTED READING

Dripps R, ed. Introduction to anesthesia. 5th ed. Philadelphia: WB Saunders, 1977:149.

Goodman L, Gilman A, eds. The pharmacological basis of therapeutics. 5th ed. New York: MacMillan, 1975:81.

Rodman M, Smith D. Clinical pharmacology in nursing. 1st ed. Philadelphia: JB Lippincott, 1984:171.

61

PNEUMATIC ANTISHOCK TROUSERS

JEAN MASON

Purpose

To increase peripheral resistance by circumferential compression
accomplishing increase in cardiac output
To tamponade bleeding
To immobilize fractures

Indications

- Systolic blood pressure less than 80 mm Hg
- Shock-like symptoms and systolic blood pressure of 100 mm
  Hg or less
- Pelvic fracture
- Fracture of lower extremity
- Spinal shock
- Massive abdominal bleeding

Contraindications

- Pulmonary edema
- Abdominal injury with protruding viscera (may use leg compartments)
- Pregnancy (may use leg compartments)

Potential Complications

- Development of pulmonary congestion

Equipment

Pneumatic antishock garment without gauges
Foot pump
Stethoscope
Blood pressure (BP) equipment

Procedure

1. Evaluate patient (including his vital signs) and leave BP cuff on arm
2. Unfold trousers and lay them flat on a long spine board or stretcher
3. Maintaining immobility of the spine, place patient on stretcher so that top of garment is just below lowest rib
4. Wrap trousers around left leg and fasten velcro strips
5. Wrap trousers around right leg and fasten velcro strips
6. Wrap abdominal compartment around abdomen and fasten velcro strips. Be sure top of garment is below bottom ribs.
7. If foot pump is used, attach air tubes to connections of trousers. It is quicker to blow up the compartments with your mouth; if you prefer to do it this way, you do not need foot pump, air tubes, or gauges at all.
8. Recheck and record vital signs
9. Inflate leg compartments first, while monitoring BP. If BP is lower than 100–110 mm Hg, inflate abdominal compartment.
10. When the patient's BP is adequate (100–110 mg Hg), turn stopcocks to hold pressure

Follow-Up

1. Auscultate patient's chest and watch closely for signs of pulmonary edema
2. Continue monitoring patient's BP, adding pressure to trous-

ers as needed. *Remember,* it is not the pressure in the trousers you are monitoring, but the pressure in the patient.

3. Once trousers have been placed on a patient, they should be removed only under a physician's direction unless pulmonary edema develops

4. During removal there must be constant monitoring of vital signs. A BP drop of 5 mm Hg signals a halt to deflation until more fluid can be replaced.

Documentation

Initial vital signs
Continuous monitoring of vital signs
Restlessness or signs of hypoxia
Intravenous lines in place, gauge of catheter, and amount of fluid
  infused
Urinary output

SUGGESTED READING

Campbell JE. Application of military antishock trousers (MAST). In: Campbell JE, ed. Basic trauma life support: advanced prehospital care. Bowie, MD: Brady Communications, 1985.

Campbell JE. Shock. In: Campbell JE, ed. Basic trauma life support: advanced prehospital care. Bowie, MD: Brady Communications, 1985.

La Fevers S, Marshall L. Introduction to intermediate skills. In: La Fevers S, Marshall L, eds. Prehospital care for the EMT—intermediate: assessment and intervention. Virginia: Reston Publishing, 1984.

Rothstein RJ. Hemorrhagic shock in multiple trauma. In: Meislin HW, ed. Priorities in multiple trauma. Germantown, MD: Aspen Publishing, 1980:29.

62

HYPERTHERMIC PATIENT TREATMENT

NANCY WEINBERG

Purpose

To reduce the patient's core temperature to 38.9 °C (102 °F) within 30 minutes to 1 hour

Indications

- Elevated core temperature greater than 38.9 °C due to heat exposure

Contraindications

- None

Potential Complications

- Hypothermia
- Hypotension
- Dysrhythmias
- Vasoconstriction
- Shivering

Equipment

Tub
Ice

Rectal thermometer with rectal probe
Intravenous (IV) normal saline
IV tubing
Large bore intracaths
Laboratory tubes
Tourniquet
Heparinized arterial blood gas syringe
Endotracheal tube
Laryngoscope
Stylet
Cardiac monitor
Cardiac arrest cart
Diazepam
Phenothiazine
Large gastric lavage tube
Iced saline for lavage

Procedure

1. Establish airway; if patient is comatose, assist physician with endotracheal intubation (see *Endotracheal Intubation*)
2. Establish IV of normal saline with a large bore intracath, administer slowly
3. Remove clothing
4. Insert rectal probe into rectum approximately 4–6 inches
5. Apply cardiac monitor
6. Monitor vital signs q15min
7. Initiate cooling process immediately by:
   a) Immersing patient in ice water tub
   b) Briskly massaging immersed patient
8. Obtain baseline laboratories which include:
   a) Arterial blood gas
   b) Complete blood count
   c) Platelets

d) CPK
e) SGOT
f) Blood urea nitrogen
g) Creatinine
h) Electrolytes
i) Bilirubin
j) Prothrombin time
k) Serum lactate
l) Amylase

9. Place indwelling Foley catheter, monitor urine output
10. Administer 500 ml of IV normal saline at rapid rate if patient is hypotensive
11. Administer IV pressors as ordered for refractory hypotension
12. Administer IV diazepam (Valium) as ordered for suppression of seizure activity
13. Administer IV phenothiazine as ordered for shivering
14. Continue to monitor core temperature with rectal probe. Continue cooling process to a core temperature of 38.9°C.
15. Assist physician with iced saline gastric lavage

Follow-Up

1. Monitor core temperature for increase in core temperature
2. Anticipate underlying disease processes
3. Anticipate tissue injury and complications

Documentation

Pretreatment assessment
Treatment provided
Duration of treatment
Patient response to treatment—special emphasis should be given to temperature and potential for tissue injury
Medications administered

SUGGESTED READING

Anderson R. The spectrum of environmental heat illness. Parkland Internal Medicine Grand Rounds 1983.

Callaham M. Heat illness. In: Rosen P, Baker FJ II, Braer GH, Dailey RH, Levy RG, eds. Emergency medicine concepts and clinical practice. Vol. I. Saint Louis: CV Mosby, 1983:477.

Smith J. Summer hazards, heatstroke. Drug Ther 1987; August.

63

HYPOTHERMIC PATIENT TREATMENT

NANCY WEINBERG

Purpose

To increase patient's core temperature to greater than 35 °C at an approximate rate of 0.55 °C per hour

Indications

- Core temperature of less than 35 °C

Contraindications

- None

Potential Complications

- Cardiac arrest
- Arrhythmias
- Ventricular fibrillation
- "Rewarming shock"
- Increased lactic acidosis

Equipment

Cardiac arrest cart
Cardiac monitor
Rectal thermometer with probe

Intravenous (IV) solutions of various kinds
Warmed blankets
Hot water bottles
Hot water mattress
Warmed saline and water for lavage procedure
Peritoneal lavage tray
Colonic lavage kit
Gastric lavage kit
Blood warmers (utilized to warm IV solutions)
Radiant head cradle
Heated oxygen
Dialysis equipment

Procedure

1. Establish airway; if patient is comatose, assist physician with endotracheal intubation
2. Remove clothing
3. Apply cardiac monitor
4. Assess patient's status
5. Obtain complete vital signs. Core temperature should be obtained by using a rectal thermometer. Insert probe into rectum and advance approximately 4–6 inches.
6. Initiate IV line with dextrose and water at keep open rate
7. Apply supplemental oxygen
8. Obtain blood samples for laboratory studies. Samples should include the following:
   a) Complete blood count
   b) Platelets
   c) Glucose
   d) BUN and creatinine
   e) Electrolytes
   f) Bicarbonate
   g) Amylase

h) Arterial blood gas

i) Urinalysis

j) Prothrombin time

k) Partial thromboplastin time

9. Obtain the following blood samples if indicated by the physician:

a) Serum lactate

b) Serum ketones

c) Toxicology screen

d) Carboxyhemoglobin

e) Calcium

f) Magnesium

g) Inorganic phosphate

h) Cortisol

i) Thyroxine

j) CPK

10. If patient's core temperature is greater than 32 °C but less than 35 °C, initiate passive external warming techniques:

a) Apply warmed blankets

11. If patient's core temperature is less than 32 °C:

a) Insert indwelling urinary catheter and monitor urine output

b) Monitor complete vital signs

c) Initiate and/or assist with active external and internal warming techniques

Active External Warming Techniques

(1) Hot water bottles applied to body surface

(2) Immersion of patient into 40 °C bath

(3) Application of hot water mattress

Active Internal Warming Techniques

(1) Warmed IV solution

(2) Warmed gastric lavage

(3) Warmed peritoneal lavage

(4) Warmed colonic lavage

      (5) Heated oxygen
      (6) Radiant heat cradle applied over torso
      (7) Warmed mediastinal lavage
      (8) Hemodialysis
12. Administer medication as ordered
13. Continue monitoring of patient. Be prepared to resuscitate patient. No hypothermic patient should be pronounced dead by physician until the core temperature is above 30°C.

Follow-Up

1. Continue to monitor patient's:
   a) Core temperature
   b) Vital signs
   c) Cardiac rhythm
   d) Urine output
   e) Mental status
2. Continue warming techniques until patient's core temperature is greater than 35°C

Documentation

Patient assessment
Core temperature
Vital signs
Cardiac rhythm
Urine output
Passive external warming techniques
Patient's response
Any medications administered
Pertinent laboratory data

SUGGESTED READING

Danzel DF. Accidental hypothermia. In: Rosen P, Baker FJ II, Braer GH, Dailey RH, Levy RC, eds. Emergency medicine concepts and clinical practice. Vol. I. Saint Louis: CV Mosby, 1983:477.

O'Keefe KM. Treatment of accidental hypothermia and rewarming techniques. In: Roberts JR, Hedges JR, eds. Clinical procedures in emergency medicine. Philadelphia: WB Saunders, 1985:1040.

Reed G. Emergency: accidental hypothermia. Hosp Med 1984; 20:13–42.

II

ASSESSMENT GUIDELINES

64

CARDIAC ASSESSMENT

MOLLY A. SEAMAN

Purpose

To assess patients who have cardiac complaints

Indications

- Patients with:
  - Chest pain
  - Arrhythmias
  - Shortness of breath
  - Trauma to chest
  - History of cardiovascular disease
- As a baseline assessment during patient admission

Equipment

Stethoscope
Electrodes
Electrocardiogram (ECG) monitor with printout
Sphygmomanometer
Calipers (optional)

Procedure

1. Gather equipment at bedside
2. If patient is awake, explain all procedures carefully
3. Provide as comfortable, private, and quiet a place as possible

4. Ensure that airway, breathing, and circulation are maintained prior to beginning assessment
5. Inquire from patient or family the nature of chief complaint
6. Have patient and/or family describe any signs or symptoms that may be present
7. Investigate presence of pain for onset, severity, location, duration, and what, if any, activity aggravates or relieves pain. (Other symptoms should be investigated as well.)
8. Obtain current and past medical history. In addition, note the use of any medication, drugs, or alcohol.
9. Record baseline data to include pulse, blood pressure, respiratory rate, and temperature. Obtain pulse and blood pressure with patient in supine and standing positions (if patient's condition does not contraindicate it). Note level of consciousness.
10. Assess peripheral pulses for presence, rhythm, and character
11. While checking pulses, observe skin for temperature, turgor, color, and moisture. Note any edema.
12. Next, observe chest for appearance, pulsations, symmetry, and injuries. At this time, observe neck for presence of pulsations and/or distention from internal jugular veins. This is best done with patient at a 45 degree angle.
13. Next, palpate point of maximum intensity (PMI). This represents the location of the left ventricle and can usually be palpated at the 5th intercostal space near the midclavicular line. The PMI may shift positions due to hypertrophy.
14. With stethoscope, auscultate heart for normal and abnormal sounds. Listen over the five auscultation points (Fig. 64–1):
    a) Aortic area: right 2nd intercostal space
    b) Pulmonary: left 2nd intercostal space
    c) Tricuspid area: 5th intercostal space close to the sternum
    d) Mitral area: left 5th intercostal space near mid clavicular line

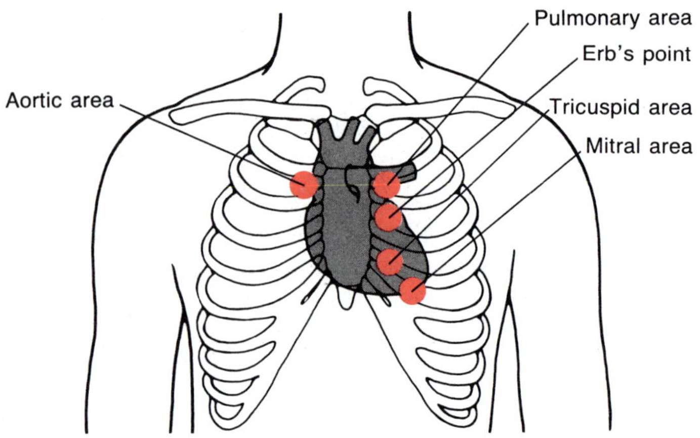

Figure 64–1   Five auscultation points for heart sounds.

     e) Erb's point: left 3rd intercostal space

15. Use the diaphragm of stethoscope to pick up high pitch sounds (such as S_1 and S_2) and the bell to hear the lower pitch sounds (such as S_3, S_4, and some murmurs).

16. If not already done, place electrodes on patient to monitor cardiac rhythm

17. Run strip off monitor (at least a 6-inch strip)

18. Check rhythm strip noting rate, rhythm, presence of P waves, duration of PR interval, duration of QRS interval, and appearance of T waves. The calipers can be used to measure the R-R interval. A piece of paper can also be used marking the R-R interval.

19. Do a 12-lead ECG (for an even closer assessment of cardiac function) if ordered by physician

Follow-Up

1. Repeat vital signs as indicated
2. Continue to monitor rhythm
3. Position patient as indicated for comfort

Documentation

Chief complaint and presence of any signs and symptoms
Pertinent patient medical history and current medications
Vital signs on admission, noting any change from supine to lying
  position
Presence or absence of pulses as well as their character
Color, temperature, turgor, and moisture of skin
General appearance of chest and any abnormalities
Any jugular vein distention
Location of PMI
Presence of normal and abnormal heart sounds
Attach a small strip of initial rhythm strip. Record rhythm and
  any abnormalities noted.

SUGGESTED READING

Bates B. The heart. In: Bates B, ed. A guide to physical exam. Philadelphia: JB Lippincott, 1974:112.

Harvey M. Patient assessment. In: Michaelson CM, ed. Congestive heart failure. Saint Louis: CV Mosby, 1983:134.

Yacone LA. Cardiac assessment. RN 1987;5:43–48.

65

NEUROLOGIC ASSESSMENT

KAREN KRENTZ

Purpose

To identify and assess patients who have neurologic abnormalities

Indications

- Patients presenting with suspected neurologic abnormalities

Equipment

Neurologic record
Penlight

Procedure

1. Assess airway patency, breathing, and circulation and intervene if necessary
2. The quickest sensitive test of neurologic status is the level of consciousness. Determine status by response to verbal and tactile stimuli. Subsequently, by more detailed examination of pupillary, respiratory, and motor reflexes. This can be correlated to the Glasgow Coma Score (Table 65–1).
   a) Observe degree of stimulus required to elicit eye opening:
      (1) Opening spontaneously—patient opens eyes without stimulus
      (2) Opening to speech—patient opens eyes to verbal stimuli (this may not be considered response to commands)

(3) Opening to pain—patient opens eyes to deep pain (this may be elicited by applying pressure to the nail bed)

(4) No eye opening—no eye opening to any stimuli (this implies marked neurologic depression)

b) Observe patient's best verbal response:

(1) Oriented speech—correctly acknowledges person, place, and time. (Keep in mind that the emergency department patient may be unsure of their exact location or time of day.)

(2) Confused conversation—although able to carry on a conversation, the patient may not produce appropriate answers to questions (i.e., person, place, time)

(3) Inappropriate words—patient exclaims simple words (often obscenities or names) at random, but does not answer questions

TABLE 65–1 Glasgow Coma Scale

1.	Eye opening:	
	Spontaneous	4
	To voice	3
	To pain	2
	None	1
2.	Verbal response:	
	Oriented	5
	Confused	4
	Inappropriate words	3
	Incomprehensible sounds	2
	None	1
3.	Motor response:	
	Obeys commands	6
	Localizes (pain)	5
	Withdraw (pain)	4
	Flexion (pain)	3
	Extension (pain)	2
	None	1

Total GCS Point (1 + 2 + 3)

(4) Uncomprehensible sounds—consists of moans or mumbles

(5) No verbal response—no verbal response to prolonged stimuli

c) Assess best motor response to stimuli (this includes assessment of each extremity as response may vary):

(1) Obeys commands—obeys commands appropriately

(2) Localizes to pain—patient responds purposefully in attempt to remove painful stimuli.

(3) Semipurposeful—patient responds to pain by grimacing or moving, but is unable to locate or remove painful stimuli

(4) Abnormal flexion—abnormal response to pain, when patient flexes arms towards shoulders and wrists are internally rotated

(5) Abnormal extension—extension response to painful stimuli, when patient's elbows straighten and shoulders internally rotate

(6) Flaccid or flicker—little or no response to pain despite repeated painful stimuli

NOTE: Ocular, verbal, and motor response should be observed simultaneously

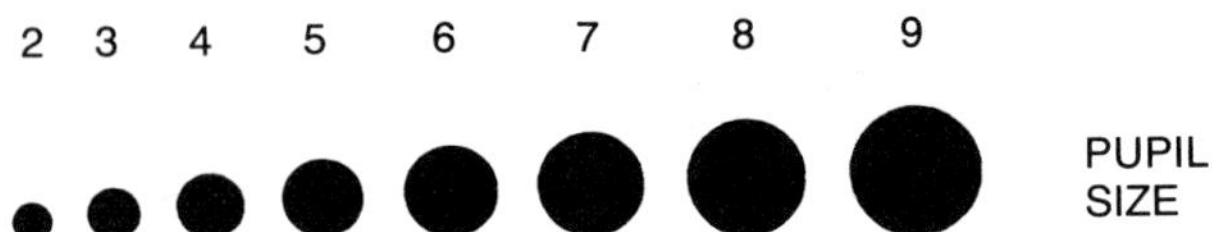

Figure 65–1 Pupil size chart.

3. Evaluate pupils:
   a) Compare size and shape of each pupil to each other and a standardized chart measured in millimeters (see Fig. 65–1).
   b) Dim lights and approach each pupil with a penlight. Evaluate each eye for pupillary constriction. Look for brisk, sluggish, or nonreactive pupils.
   c) Unusual eye movements such as nystagmus or dysconjugate gaze may be observed

4. Evaluate extremities separately right and left, upper and lower (response of each must be charted separately if findings are not bilateral):
   a) Normal power—patient's limbs have normal strength
   b) Can overcome resistance—patient's limbs are weak, but can overcome resistance applied by examiner
   c) Cannot overcome resistance—patient may have weak functioning of the extremity, but cannot overcome resistance
   d) Overcomes gravity—patient's limbs cannot overcome resistance, but can, even if momentarily, raise extremity off bed
   e) Flicker of muscle—muscle movement may be seen or felt, but patient is unable to move extremity
   f) None—extremity is flaccid and does not respond to stimulation

5. Evaluate basic protective reflexes:
   a) Corneal reflex—stimulation causes a bilateral blink and upward deviation of eyes
   b) Gag reflex—absence indicates inability to handle secretions

6. Evaluate vital signs (changes are often noted late in neurologic deterioration):
   a) Respirations—rate, depth, and regularity are observed. A specific description of respirations should be document-

ed rather than attempting to identify a specific respiratory pattern.

b) Heart rate—bradycardia is observed as intracranial pressure increases. In adults, shock and the expected tachycardia is not caused by intracranial hemorrhage.

c) Blood pressure—a widened pulse pressure and hypertension are seen with increasing intracranial pressure. As with the heart rate, hypotension in the patient with neurologic deficits often indicates another source of bleeding.

d) Temperature—neurologic damage often supresses temperature control mechanisms. Therefore, patients are often hyperthermic.

Follow-Up

1. Reevaluation of neurologic status and comparison to the patient's baseline must be done according to the patient's condition

Documentation

Details of initial examination
Any changes in neurologic status over time

SUGGESTED READING

Nursing policy and procedure manual. Dallas: Parkland Memorial Hospital, 1986. Policy #6011–32–02.

Selfridge J. Head trauma. In: Rea R, ed. Trauma nursing core course manual. Chicago: Award Printing Corp, 1987:V–01.

Tyson GW, Rimel RW, Jane JA. Head injuries. In: Kravis TC, Warner CG, eds. Emergency medicine: a comprehensive review. 2nd ed. Rockville, MD: Aspen, 1986:831.

66

RESPIRATORY ASSESSMENT

MOLLY A. SEAMAN

Purpose

To assess patients who have respiratory complaints

Indications

- Patients with:
  - Chest pain
  - Shortness of breath
  - Chest trauma
  - History of respiratory illness or disease
- As a baseline assessment during patient admission

Equipment

Stethoscope

Procedure

1. Gather equipment at bedside
2. If patient is awake, explain all procedures carefully
3. Provide as comfortable, private, and quiet a place as possible
4. Ensure that airway, breathing and circulation are maintained prior to beginning the assessment
5. Inquire from patient and/or family member nature of chief complaint

6. If possible, have patient and/or family describe any signs or symptoms that may be present

7. The presence of pain should be investigated for onset, severity, location, duration, and what, if any, activity aggravates or relieves the pain. Other symptoms should be investigated as well.

8. Obtain current and past medical history. In addition, note the use of any medications, drugs, or alcohol.

9. Inquire from patient whether he/she is a smoker. If so, for how long and how much on a daily basis to determine pack years.

10. Record baseline data, to include pulse, blood pressure, respiratory rate, and temperature. Level of consciousness should be noted.

11. Observe patient for general appearance. Is patient thin or obese? What is the color, temperature, and moisture of skin? Is there any cyanosis present?

12. Observe chest for symmetry, appearance, trauma, or movement. What muscles are used during respiration? Are there sternal retractions. Does patient lean forward to breathe better? Does patient appear short of breath?

13. Palpate anterior and posterior thorax for tenderness

14. If patient's condition permits, percuss thorax to detect any abnormal air, fluid, or masses present

15. Next, auscultate patient's lungs. This is best done with patient sitting; however, if condition does not allow this, auscultate with patient in supine position.

16. Have patient breathe through his mouth taking normal, but deeper breaths

17. With stethoscope, listen from side to side anteriorly and posteriorly. Begin at apex of lungs working down to bases (Fig. 66-1).

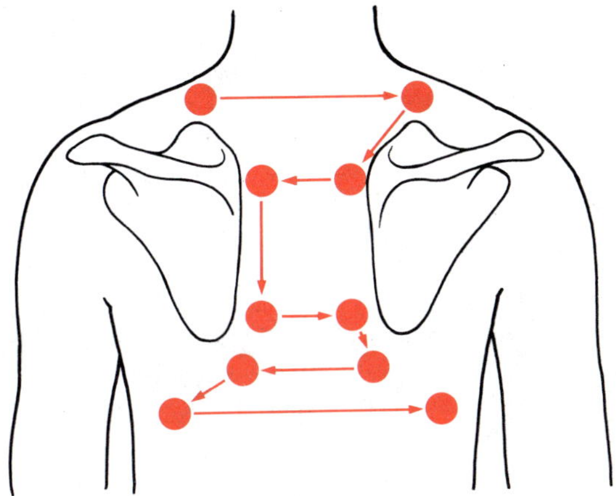

Figure 66–1 Sequence of posterior examination of lungs.

Follow-Up

1. The physician may order further tests to assist in determining respiratory status. Tests, such as the pulmonary function test (PFT), assist in determining lung volumes and airway problems. An arterial blood gas (ABG) may also be ordered. Depending on the facility, the nurse may or may not perform this function. The ABG assists in determining oxygenation, pH, and ventilation status. Additionally, a bronchoscopy may be ordered diagnostically or therapeutically. The nurse should assist the physician and explain any procedures carefully.

2. Continue to monitor patient's respiratory status before and after treatments

Documentation

Initial respiratory rate, noting the rhythm and use of accessory muscles

Any obvious deformities, sternal retractions, injuries, or cyanosis

The position in which the patient can best breathe

Any pain that the patient may have or that is felt upon palpation

The presence of normal or abnormal breath sounds and their location

Presence and location of any abnormal sounds, if percussion is done

Whether or not patient smokes, along with how much and how often

Any cough or shortness of breath

SUGGESTED READING

Bates B. The thorax and lungs. In: Bates B, ed. A guide to physical exam. Philadelphia: JB Lippincott, 1974:81.

Simoneau, J. Patient assessment. In: Barber J, Sheehy SB, eds. Saint Louis: CV Mosby, 1985:106.

Woody JW, Egger S, Gyetvan M. Collecting and assessing patient data. In: Robinson J, ed. Providing respiratory care. Nursing 80. Horsham, PA: Intermed Communications, 1979:10.

67

TRAUMA ASSESSMENT

KAREN KRENTZ

Purpose

To identify and assess patients presenting with traumatic injuries

Indications

- Patients who present with suspected traumatic injuries

Equipment

Penlight
Trauma Record

Procedure

1. **Perform primary survey:**
   The primary survey is the initial assessment by emergency care personnel. Life-threatening conditions are identified first, and simultaneous management is begun:
   a) Airway maintenance and cervical spine immobilization are the first priorities of trauma care. Attempts to maintain a patent airway begin with the jaw thrust-chin lift and the removal of blood, vomitus, or other debris to clear the airway. The type of airway needed is determined by the patient's respiratory status. An oral or nasal airway is appropriate if the airway has not been seriously compromised. Endotracheal intubation or cricothyrotomy is

indicated if a patent airway cannot be maintained. Special attention is given to potential cervical spine injuries and prevention of further damage by avoiding hyperflexion or hyperextension of the neck.

b) Assess the patient's breathing by feeling for air movement from the mouth and nose. The patient's chest is exposed to observe for adequate respiratory efforts. Watch the patient's attempts to breathe and observe the chest for bilateral symmetric expansion. Examine the chest for obvious injury to the chest wall. Auscultate for breath sounds or the *sucking* sound of an open chest wall. If the patient has inadequate respirations, artificial ventilatory assistance is started with a bag-valve device and high flow oxygen. If respirations are present, they should be assessed for rate and depth. Cyanosis and decreased level of consciousness indicate poor oxygenation. Special attention is given to these life-threatening injuries:

(1) *Tension pneumothorax:*

Occurs when free air in the pleural space increases to the point where the lung collapses, mediastinal structures are displaced, and the heart and great vessels are compressed. Symptoms include respiratory distress, tracheal deviation and mediastinal shift away from the affected side, and neck vein distention. This increasing pressure must be relieved by needle thoracotomy and chest tube insertion.

(2) *Sucking chest wound:*

Is caused by air entering the thoracic cavity through an open chest wound. The tell tale ''sucking'' noise can be heard at the entrance of the chest wound as air is drawn into the chest. To prevent further pneumothorax, the wound is covered with vasoline gauze and a sterile dressing. Continued observation for tension pneumothorax is important.

(3) *Flail chest:*

Is exhibited by paradoxical movement of the chest wall with respiratory difficulty. A group of ribs with multiple fractures may be found, which causes instability in the chest wall. Inability to ventilate the patient poses a significant management problem. High risk patients, such as those with pulmonary contusion often require mechanical ventilation.

(4) *Hemothorax:*

Caused by hemorrhage from intrapleural or interstitial injury and may display symptoms of respiratory difficulty from inadequate lung expansion. Should bleeding continue, shock from hypovolemia occurs. Blood must be removed from the chest via a large bore chest tube. Occasionally, surgical repair may be needed to obtain hemostasis.

c) Cardiac output is assessed initially by palpating the pulse for intensity, quality, and regularity. A blood pressure reading may be optional until the primary survey is complete. Presence of a palpable peripheral pulse indicates a systolic blood pressure of at least 80 mm Hg. The pulseless victim requires initiation of cardiac life support. Exsanguinating hemorrhage should be identified and controlled in the primary survey. Direct pressure, pneumatic splints, and the pneumatic antishock garment may be helpful. Volume replacement begins immediately with crystalloid solution via at least two large bore intravenous catheters. Blood samples for hematocrit and type and crossmatch should be sent. Uncrossmatched type specific blood and/or autotransfusion may be used in severe hemorrhage with shock.

2. **Perform brief neurologic examination:**

A rapid neurologic evaluation is done at the end of the primary survey. This examination should establish patient's level of consciousness and response to stimuli. Pupillary size and reaction are also observed. This examination may determine need for neurosurgical intervention. (See *Neurologic Assessment.*)

3. **Perform secondary survey:**

   At this point the patient is undressed totally and an organ systems assessment is begun. A change in the primary assessment may require immediate intervention at any time.

   a) The skull and face are examined for obvious injuries such as fractures, surface trauma, or impaled objects. Eyes should be checked for extraocular movements, visual changes, and subconjunctival hemorrhage. Pupils are reevaluated for response and size. The ears and nose are evaluated for bleeding or cerebral spinal leak. The patient's mouth should be examined for broken teeth or malocclusion.

   b) The neck should be palpated and visualized after complete immobilization. Observe for trauma, tracheal deviation, edema, airway patency, and distended neck veins. Palpate for point tenderness along the cervical spine and for cutaneous emphysema. Simultaneous intervention includes maintenance of cervical spine immobilization, reevaluation of the airway, and x-ray films.

   c) Observe the chest for surface trauma, paradoxical chest wall movement, and costal retractions. Palpate for point tenderness, fractures, and crepitus. Auscultate for diminished or absent breath sounds and distant or abnormal heart sounds. Recheck pulses and respiratory efforts for changes from the primary assessment. Evaluate blood pressure and monitor cardiac rhythm. Other diagnostic procedures should include chest x-ray film, 12-lead electrocardiogram, arterial blood gases, and monitoring blood loss.

d) The abdomen should be inspected for surface trauma, entrance and exit wounds, and distention. Auscultate bowel sounds in four quadrants prior to palpation. Palpation of the abdomen may reveal rigidity, guarding, rebound tenderness, and pain. The patient with suspected abdominal injury and altered level of consciousness may require peritoneal lavage, computerized tomography, or exploratory laparotomy to rule out intra-abdominal injury. A nasogastric tube is inserted to check gastric aspirate for blood. Urethral catheterization for urinalysis and observation for gross hematuria assists in the evaluation of genitourinary injuries.

e) Observe for soft tissue edema, hematoma, or suprapubic mass of the pelvis and genitalia. Palpate the pelvis for bony instability. A rectal exam is done to assess for bleeding, location of the prostate, and sphincter tone. Observe for testicular trauma, and look for blood at the tip of the penile meatus.

f) Evaluate extremities for musculoskeletal injuries by inspecting for contusions or deformity. Palpate for point tenderness or crepitus. Other indications of musculoskeletal trauma include decreased strength, false motion, and swelling. It is important to reevaluate extremities frequently for color, movement, and sensation. Peripheral pulses and skin color should be compared. Potential fractures are splinted, immobilized, and evaluated by x-ray film. Continued assessment for blood loss and possibly pain medication should be considered.

g) Each trauma patient must be log rolled and examined posteriorly. The patient's back is evaluated for the same abnormalities as noted in secondary assessment. Frequently, injuries are overlooked and treatment delayed by failing to adequately examine the back.

h) A neurologic reevaluation of level of consciousness and pupillary size and reaction is important. Then a more in-depth neurologic exam including motor and sensory response of extremities is done. Quantification of deficits by standardized numeric evaluation, such as the Glasgow Coma Score facilitates early recognition of changes in neurologic status.

4. **Calculate trauma score:**

The trauma score is an assessment tool composed of respiratory rate and expansion, systolic blood pressure, capillary refill, and neurologic response. It numerically identifies the physiologic status of the trauma victim. This information may be done in the prehospital setting and its changes documented throughout the resuscitation of the patient (Table 67–1 and 2).

5. **Obtain complete patient history:**

The patient's pertinent history should be obtained by interviews with the patient, family, or prehospital personnel. Past medical history, including current illnesses and past operations are documented. Allergies, especially to medications, should be readily available on the chart. Medications, both prescription and over-the-counter, are to be noted. Alcohol and abused drugs need to be included. Always determine the amount of alcohol or drugs ingested and the time of last usage. For patients in need of surgical intervention, find out when and what was the last oral intake. Finally, try to determine the precipitating events or cause of the traumatic injury. Information regarding circumstances and weapons used may be helpful in determining the extent of injury. Always include the patient's condition at the scene and prehospital treatment rendered in your documentation.

Table 67–1   Calculation of a Trauma Score[*]

The Trauma Score is a numerical grading system for estimating the severity of injury. The score is composed of the Glasgow Coma Scale (reduced to approximately one-third total value) and measurements of cardiopulmonary function. Each parameter is given a number (high for normal and low for impaired function). Severity of injury is estimated by summing the numbers. The lowest score is 1, and the highest is 16.

Respiratory rate	10–24/min	4
	24–35/min	3
	36/min or greater	2
	1–9/min	1
	None	0
Respiratory expansion	Normal	1
	Retractive (use of accessory muscles or intercostal retraction)	0
Systolic blood pressure (auscultate or palpate either arm)	90 mm Hg or greater	4
	70–89 mm Hg	3
	50–69 mm Hg	2
	0–49 mm Hg	1
	No carotid pulse	0
Capillary refill (nailbed, forehead, or lip mucosa)	Normal	2
	Delayed (more than 2 seconds)	1
	None	0

Glasgow Coma Scale

Eye opening	Spontaneous	4	Total Glasgow Coma Scale Points		
	To voice	3			
	To pain	2	14–15	=	5
	None	1	11–13	=	4
Best verbal response (to voice or or painful stimulus)	Oriented	5	8 –10	=	3
	Confused	4	5 – 7	=	2
	Inappropriate words	3	3 – 4	=	1
	Incomprehensible words	2			
	None	1			
Best motor response (to command or painful stimulus)	Obeys command	6			
	Localizes pain	5			
	Withdraw (pain)	4			
	Flexion (pain)	3			
	Extension (pain)	2			
	None	1			

Total Trauma Score	1–16

[*] Endorsed by the American Trauma Society (From Champion HR, Sacco WJ, Carnazzo AJ, et al. Trauma score. Crit Care Med 1981;9(9):672–676.)

Table 67–2 Projected Estimate of Survival for Each Value of the Trauma Score Based on 1,059 Patients with Blunt Penetrating Injury

Trauma Score	Percentage Survival
16	99
15	98
14	96
13	93
12	87
11	76
10	60
9	42
8	26
7	15
6	8
5	4
4	2
3	1
2	0
1	0

From Champion HR, Sacco WH, et al. Trauma score. Crit Care Med 1981; 9(9):672–676.

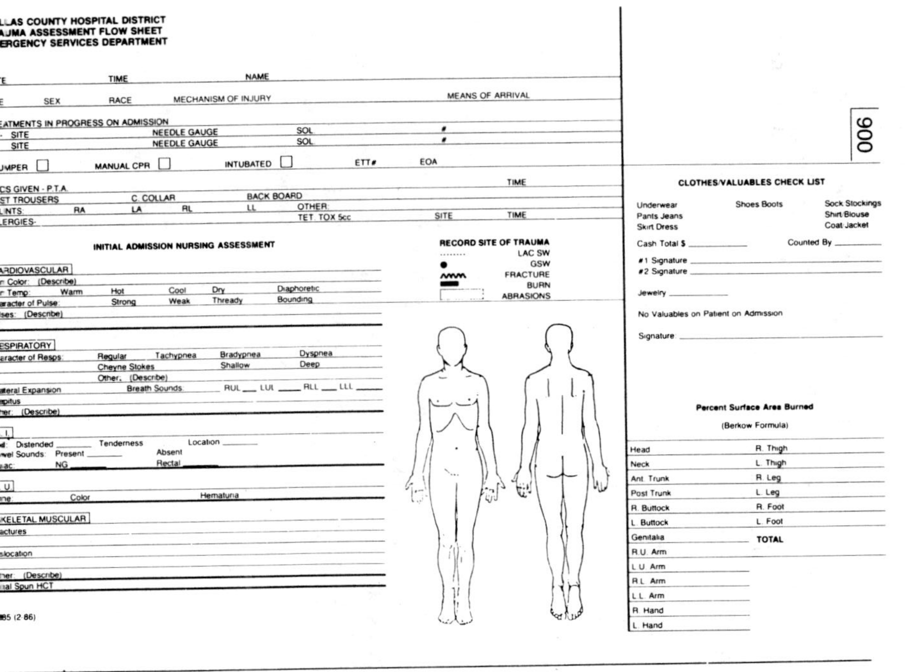

Figure 67–1 Trauma assessment flow sheet, emergency services department, Dallas County Hospital District.

Follow-Up

1. Reevaluation and comparison to the patient's baseline must be done according to the patient's condition
2. Frequent nursing assessment is indicated in the trauma patient

Documentation

Details of initial examination (Fig. 67–1)
Any changes in patient status over time
Past medical history
History of precipitating event

SUGGESTED READING

Colicot E, et al. Advanced trauma life support student manual. American College of Surgeons, 1984:5.

Hall MM. Initial assessment. In: Rea R, ed. Trauma nursing care course manual. Chicago: Emergency Nurses Association, 1987:III–1.

Jacobs LM, Bennett B. Management of the multisystem–injured patient. In: Kravis TC, ed. Emergency medicine. A comprehensive review. 2nd ed. Rockville, MD: Aspen, 1987:63.

III

APPENDICES

A
____

AMERICAN HEART ASSOCIATION ADVANCED CARDIAC LIFE SUPPORT ALGORITHMS

MARY E. MANCINI

These sequences were developed to assist in teaching how to treat a broad range of patients. Some patients may require care not specified herein. These algorithms should not be construed as prohibiting such flexibility. These algorithms are adapted from the American Heart Association. Standards and guidelines for cardiopulmonary resuscitation and emergency care. JAMA June 6, 1986; 255 (21) 2841–3044.

Figure 1 Ventricular fibrillation (VF) and pulseless ventricular tachycardia (VT).

[a] Pulseless VT should be treated identically to VF.

[b] Check pulse and rhythm after each shock. If VF recurs after transiently converting (rather than persists without ever converting), use whatever energy level has previously been successful for defibrillation.

[c] Epinephrine should be repeated every five minutes.

[d] Intubation is preferable. If it can be accomplished simultaneously with other techniques, then the earlier the better. However, defibrillation and epinephrine are more important initially if the patient can be ventilated without intubation.

[e] Some may prefer repeated doses of lidocaine, which may be given in 0.5-mg/kg boluses every eight minutes to a total dose of 3 mg/kg.

[f] Value of sodium bicarbonate is questionable during cardiac arrest, and it is not recommended for routine cardiac arrest sequence. Consideration of its use in a dose of 1 mEq/kg is appropriate at this point. Half of original dose may be repeated every ten minutes if it is used.

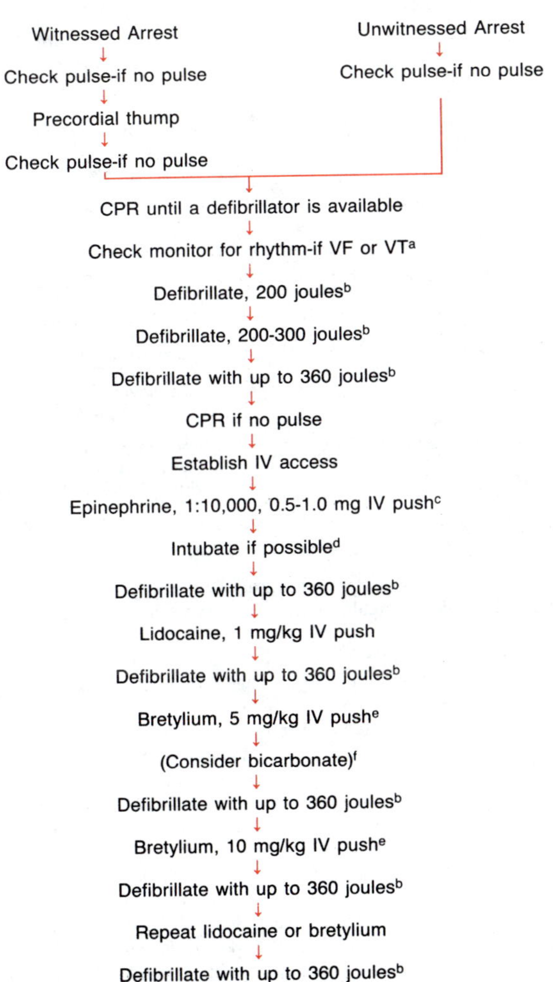

Witnessed Arrest
Check pulse-if no pulse
Precordial thump
Check pulse-if no pulse
Unwitnessed Arrest
Check pulse-if no pulse
CPR until a defibrillator is available
Check monitor for rhythm-if VF or VT[a]
Defibrillate, 200 joules[b]
Defibrillate, 200-300 joules[b]
Defibrillate with up to 360 joules[b]
CPR if no pulse
Establish IV access
Epinephrine, 1:10,000, 0.5-1.0 mg IV push[c]
Intubate if possible[d]
Defibrillate with up to 360 joules[b]
Lidocaine, 1 mg/kg IV push
Defibrillate with up to 360 joules[b]
Bretylium, 5 mg/kg IV push[e]
(Consider bicarbonate)[f]
Defibrillate with up to 360 joules[b]
Bretylium, 10 mg/kg IV push[e]
Defibrillate with up to 360 joules[b]
Repeat lidocaine or bretylium
Defibrillate with up to 360 joules[b]

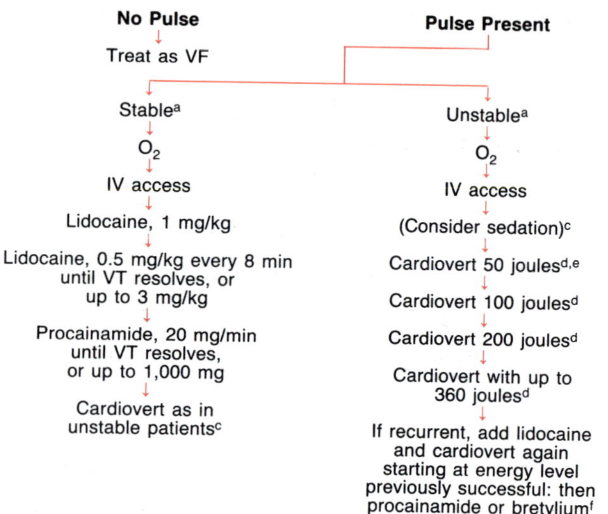

Figure 2 Sustained ventricular tachycardia (VT).

[a] If patient becomes unstable at any time, move to ''Unstable'' arm of algorithm.

[b] Unstable indicates symptoms (e.g., chest pain or dyspnea), hypotension (systolic blood pressure <90 mm Hg), congestive heart failure, ischemia, or infarction.

[c] Sedation should be considered for all patients, including those defined in footnote b as unstable, except those who are hemodynamically unstable (e.g., hypotensive, in pulmonary edema, or unconscious).

[d] If hypotension, pulmonary edema, or unconsciousness is present, unsynchronized cardioversion should be done to avoid delay associated with synchronization.

[e] In the absence of hypotension, pulmonary edema, or unconsciousness, a precordial thump may be employed prior to cardioversion.

[f] Once VT has resolved, begin intravenous (IV) infusion of antiarrhythmic agent that has aided resolution of VT. If hypotension, pulmonary edema, or unconsciousness is present, use lidocaine if cardioversion alone is unsuccessful, followed by bretylium. In all other patients, recommended order of therapy is lidocaine, procainamide, and then bretylium.

If Rhythm is Unclear and Possibly Ventricular
Fibrillation, Defibrillate as for VF. If Asystole is Present[a]

Continue CPR

Establish IV access

Epinephrine, 1:10,000, 0.5-1.0 mg IV push[b]

Intubate when possible[c]
Atropine, 1.0 mg IV push (repeated in 5 min)

(Consider bicarbonate)[d]

Consider pacing

Figure 3 Asystole (cardiac standstill).

[a] Asystole should be confirmed in two leads.

[b] Epinephrine should be repeated every five minutes.

[c] Intubation is preferable; if it can be accomplished simultaneously with other techniques, then the earlier the better. However, cardiopulmonary resuscitation (CPR) and use of epinephrine are more important initially if patient can be ventilated without intubation. (Endotracheal epinephrine may be used.)

[d] Value of sodium bicarbonate is questionable during cardiac arrest, and it is not recommended for the routine cardiac arrest sequence. Consideration of its use in a dose of 1 mEq/kg is appropriate at this point. Half of original dose may be repeated every ten minutes if it is used.

Continue CPR
↓
Establish IV access
↓
Epinephrine, 1:10,000, 0.5-1.0 mg IV push[a]
↓
Intubate when possible[b]
↓
(Consider bicarbonate)[c]
↓
Consider hypovolemia,
cardiac tamponade,
tension pneumothorax,
hypoxemia,
acidosis,
pulmonary embolism

Figure 4   Electromechanical dissociation.

[a] Epinephrine should be repeated every five minutes.

[b] Intubation is preferable. If it can be accomplished simultaneously with other techniques, then the earlier the better. However, epinephrine is more important initially if the patient can be ventilated without intubation.

[c] Value of sodium bicarbonate is questionable during cardiac arrest, and it is not recommended for routine cardiac arrest sequence. Consideration of its use in a dose of 1 mEq/kg is appropriate at this point. Half of original dose may be repeated every ten minutes if it is used.

Unstable
↓
Synchronous cardioversion 75–100 joules
↓
Synchronous cardioversion 200 joules
↓
Synchronous cardioversion 360 joules
↓
Correct underlying abnormalities
↓
Pharmacological therapy + cardioversion

Stable
↓
Vagal maneuvers
↓
Verapamil, 5 mg IV
↓
Verapamil, 10 mg IV
(in 15–20 min)
Cardioversion, digoxin,
β-Blockers, pacing as indicated

If conversion occurs but PSVT recurs, repeated electrical cardioversion is *not* indicated. Sedation should be used as time permits.

Figure 5   Paroxysmal supraventricular tachycardia (PSVT).

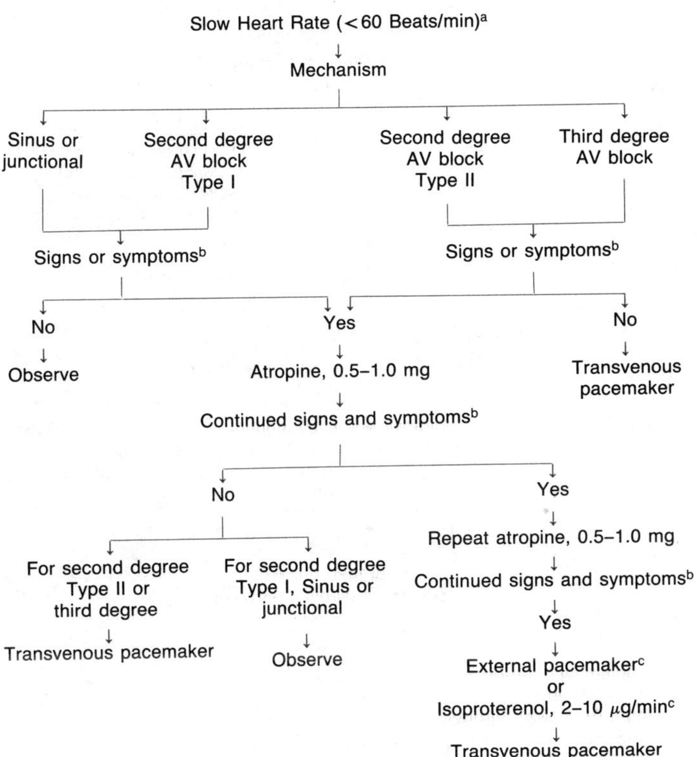

Figure 6 Bradycardia. AV indicates atrioventricular.

[a] A solitary chest thump or cough may stimulate cardiac electrical activity and result in improved cardiac output and may be used at this point.

[b] Hypotension (blood pressure <90 mm Hg), premature ventricular contractions, altered mental status or symptoms (e.g., chest pain or dyspnea), ischemia, or infarction.

[c] Temporizing therapy.

Assess for Need for
Acute Suppressive Therapy
↓

→ Rule out treatable cause
→ Consider serum potassium
→ Consider digitalis level
→ Consider bradycardia
→ Consider drugs

Lidocaine, 1 mg/kg
↓
If not suppressed,
repeat lidocaine, 0.5 mg/kg every 2–5 min,
until no ectopy, or up to 3 mg/kg given
↓
If not suppressed,
procainamide 20 mg/min
until no ectopy, or up to 1,000 mg given
↓
If not suppressed
and not contraindicated,
bretylium, 5–10 mg/kg over 8–10 min
↓
If not suppressed,
consider overdrive pacing

Once ectopy resolved, maintain as follows:
After lidocaine, 1 mg/kg...lidocaine drip, 2 mg/min
After lidocaine, 1–2 mg/kg...lidocaine drip, 3 mg/min
After lidocaine, 2–3 mg/kg...lidocaine drip, 4 mg/min
After procainamide...procainamide drip, 1–4 mg/min (Check Blood Level)
After bretylium...bretylium drip, 2 mg/min

Figure 7 Ventricular ectopy: acute suppressive therapy.

SUGGESTED READING

American Heart Association. Standards and guidelines for cardiopulmonary resuscitation and emergency care. JAMA 1986; 255(21):2841–3044.

American Heart Association. Textbook of advanced cardiac life support. 2nd ed. Dallas: American Heart Association, 1987:238.

Roth CS, Weaver DT, eds. Pocket manual of emergency medical therapy. 4th ed. Toronto: BC Decker, 1987:215.

Sheehy GB. A quick overview of the new standards and guidelines for cardiopulmonary resuscitation and emergency cardiac care. JEN 1987; 13(1):47–49.

B

BLOOD PRODUCTS

BARBARA CLARK MIMS

Blood Component	Indication(s)	Action(s)	Side Effects	Remarks
Fresh Frozen Plasma	Clotting factor deficiency when specific component unavailable, or exact factor deficiency undiagnosed	Raises level of clotting factors, produces hemostatis in bleeding patient. Increases colloidal oncotic pressure, thereby increasing intravascular volume.	Rarely, congestive heart failure	Does not contain viable platelets. Use standard blood recipient set. Volume in each unit varies and is recorded on the unit bag. Must be typed specifically for each patient but cross-matching and Rh testing are not necessary. Requires 30 minutes to thaw, so notify Blood Bank in advance.
Platelet Concentrate	Thrombocytopenia (platelet count $<20,000/mm^3$ or $<50,000/mm^3$ with active bleeding)	Raises platelet count. Produces hemostasis in bleeding patient by aiding clot formation.	Risk of transfusion transmitted diseases. May develop antibodies and destroy platelets in subsequent transfusions Risk of side effects such as chills or fever and allergic reactions are increased when multiple units of platelets are infused	Use special platelet filter. Adjust infusion rate according to volume to be delivered. Platelets are stored at room temperature with continuous rotation. *Do not* place in refrigerator.

Leukocyte-poor packed red blood cells ("Buffy-poor RBC's")	Repeated trans-fusions, renal failure, pts who have had febrile reactions to transfusions or demonstrate leukocyte anti-bodies	Raises Hgb and Hct	Same as packed red blood cells, with less risk of febrile and allergic reactions	Prepared from whole blood by removal of super-natant plasma and the "buffy coat" of leukocytes. This removes 80–90 % of total leukocytes. Requires extra preparation time.
Cryoprecipitate (Factor VIII and fibrinogen)	Hemophilia (dur-ing or in antici-pation of a bleeding episode)	Elevates factor VIII, controls bleeding in hemophiliac	Risk of transfusion transmitted diseases	Administer rapidly. Use special admin-istration set supplied by blood bank.
Plasmanate	Hypovolemia	Expands plasma volume, contains little clotting factors	Volume overload or hypotension due to vasoactive kinins with rapid infusion	Check expiration date on bottle. Heat treated to decrease risk of disease mission. Any IV tubing may be used.
Normal serum albumin	Shock, burns, hypoproteinemia	Increases colloidal oncotic pressure, thereby increasing intravascular volume	Can cause intracellular dehydration	Does not require type and cross-matching. Check expiration date on bottle. Heat treated to decrease risk of transfusion transmitted disease. Any IV tubing may be used.

SUGGESTED READING

Brunner LS, Suddarth DS, eds. The Lippincott manual of nursing practice. 3rd ed. Philadelphia: JB Lippincott, 1982:236.

Millar S, Sampson LK, Soukup M. AACN Procedure manual for critical care. Philadelphia: WB Saunders, 1985:409.

Rutman RC, Miller WV. Transfusion therapy principles and procedures. Rockville, MD: Aspen, 1982:40.

Synder EL. Blood transfusion therapy: a physician's handbook. Arlington: American Association of Blood Banks, 1983:14,25.

C

ISOLATION PROCEDURES

MARY E. MANCINI

Purpose

To prevent the spread of infectious material from one individual to another, which whould include patients, personnel, and visitors, by establishing guidelines for adequate isolation and safe handling of contaminated articles and environments (Table 1)

Techniques

- Hand Washing—Hand washing is the single most important means of preventing the spread of infection. Hand washing shall be done:
  - Before performing invasive procedures, touching wounds, or touching patients
  - After caring for an infected or colonized patient, even when gloves are used
  - After touching excretions or secretions of the infected or colonized patient
  - Between all physical patient contacts
- Mask—When masks are indicated, they shall be used only once. Discard and replace if it becomes moist. Never lower around the neck and reuse. Wash hands after removing and discarding mask. Standard high efficiency disposable masks shall be used, with the exception of respiratory and strict isolation, which require the molded high efficiency mask.

Table 1 The Most Common Emergency Department Admissions Requiring Isolation

Disease	Category	Vented Room	Private Room	Mask	Gown	Gloves
AIDS	Blood and body fluids	No	Yes	No	Sometimes (When in contact with blood and body fluids)	Sometimes (When in contact with blood and body fluids)
Cellulitis	Drainage and secretions	No	No	No	Yes	Yes
Chickenpox (Varicella)	Strict	Yes	—	Yes	Yes	Yes
Cytomegalovirus (No pregnant employees)	None	No	No	No	No	Yes
Diarrhea (Salmonella or shigella)	Enteric	No	Yes	No	Yes	Yes
Gangrene, Gas	Drainage and secretions	No	Yes	No	Yes	Yes
Rubella (No pregnant or susceptible staff)	Contact	No	Yes	Yes	Yes	Yes
Hepatitis A	Enteric	No	Yes	No	Yes	Yes
B	Blood and body fluid precautions	No	Preferably	No	Yes	Yes

Disease	Isolation					
Non A Non B	same as for A and B	No	Yes	No	Yes	Yes
Herpes Zoster	Strict	Yes	—	Yes	Yes	Yes
Malaria	Blood and body fluids	No	No	No	Sometimes	Sometimes
Measles (Rubella)	Respiratory	Yes	—	Yes	Yes	Yes
Meningitis						
Aseptic	Enteric	No	Yes	No	Yes	Yes
Bacterial	None	No	No	No	No	No
Meningococcal	Respiratory	Yes	—	Yes	No	No
Methocillin resistent Staphylococcus aureus (M.R.S.A.)	M.R.S.A. Isolation	No	Yes	No	Yes	Yes
Mumps (Parotitis)	Respiratory	Yes	—	Yes	No	No
Syphilis (primary and secondary)	Drainage, secretions, blood and body fluids	No	Yes	No	Yes	Yes
Tuberculosis						
Pulmonary	Respiratory	Yes	—	Yes	No	No
Extrapulmonary	Drainage and secretions	No	Yes	No	Yes	Yes
Viral Diseases Pericarditis Myocarditis Meningitis	Enteric	No	Yes	No	Yes	Yes

- Gowns—When gowns are indicated, they shall be worn only once and then discarded in appropriate receptacle before leaving the contaminated area. Gowns shall be available outside the patient's room or in the anteroom.
- Gloves—When gloves are indicated, disposable single-use gloves should be worn. After direct contact with a patient's excretions or secretions, gloves should be changed if care of that patient is not complete.
- Bagging of articles and linen—The double-bagging method shall be used to remove all contaminated articles and linens from the room. Double-bagging is accomplished as follows:
  - The person gowned in the room places the closed bag of contaminated articles in a clean bag held by another person outside the door
  - The outside (second) bag is closed, labeled, and appropriate disposition made. Critical to this technique is that the outside of the second bag is not touched by the person in the room or by the bag of contaminated articles.

Equipment

Disposable patient care items: Discard contaminated articles in lined waste container in patient's room

Reusable patient care items: Return double-bagged, labeled, contaminated articles to appropriate department for decontamination and reprocessing

Needles and syringes: Discard all needles and syringes in disposal containers located in patient's room. DO NOT RECAP, CUT, OR BREAK NEEDLES.

Unit equipment (sphygmomanometer, stethoscope, etc.): Clean with germicidal solution after use

Thermometers: Each patient in isolation shall be given an individual glass thermometer, which shall remain at the bedside, stored in a dry holder. These are returned to Sterile Processing Department for terminal cleaning.

Linen: Take in only amount of clean linen needed to provide patient care. Contaminated linens shall be placed in water-soluble bags in the room. On removal from room, water-soluble bags shall be placed in a laundry bag using double-bagging technique. Once secured in the second bag, label with *isolation* tape before sending to Linen Services.

Scales: After use, clean with germicidal solution

Dishes: Disposable trays shall be used to serve all meals. Disposable dishes, utensils, and trays shall be discarded by double-bagging.

Dressing and facial tissue shall be disposed of by double-bagging

Transporting Infected or Colonized Patients

Patients shall be taken out of their rooms only for essential purposes. Appropriate barriers (mask, gown, dressing) to prevent transmission shall be used by the patient and the transport person. Patients in *Strict* or *Respiratory* isolation shall wear a molded mask.

Nursing shall alert the receiving area or department of the diagnosis, category of isolation (i.e., Strict, Blood and Body Fluid Precautions, Enteric, etc.), and procedures to be followed to prevent the spread of infection. Additionally, the patient's chart shall be labeled on the front with *isolation* tag.

Clothing

Patient's clothing shall be bagged and sent home when possible. The person taking the clothing shall be instructed to wash it with detergent and hot water. Bleach should be added when possible.

SUGGESTED READING

Callaham ML, ed. Current therapy in emergency medicine. Toronto: BC Decker, 1987:777,1020.

Nursing policy and procedure manual. Dallas: Parkland Memorial Hospital, 1987. Policy #6011(17/01).

Roth CS, Weaver T, eds. Pocket manual of emergency medical therapy. 4th ed. Toronto: BC Decker, 1987:142.

D

INTRAVENOUS MEDICATION ADMINISTRATION

KAREN KRENTZ and BARBARA KALO

Drug	Indications and Primary Effects	Dose	Preparation	Special Considerations
Aminocaproic acid (Amicar)	Hemostatic (arrests the flow of blood) Indicated in severe bleeding from hyperfibrinolysis	5 g slow IV infusion, then 1–1.25 g hourly until bleeding controlled	5 g in 500 ml D5W or 18 g in 1,000 ml D5W at 83 ml/hr	1. Monitor heart rate, rhythm, and blood pressure 2. May be used as an antidote for streptokinase toxicity 3. Contraindicated in active intravascular clotting
Aminophylline	Relaxes smooth muscle of bronchial airways and pulmonary blood vessels	250–500 mg	Dilute in 100–200 ml D5W	1. IV rate not to exceed 35 mg/min
Atropine	Decreases vagal tone in pronounced bradycardia	0.5 mg IV bolus	1 mg/ml or 1 mg/10ml	1. May repeat every 5 min, up to a total dose of 2 mg
Bretylium (Bretylol)	Antiarrhythmic To treat ventricular fibrillation and tachycardia	Bolus of 5 mg/kg IV push—increase dose to 10 mg/kg infuse at 1–4 mg/min	Dilute 2 g in 500 ml D5W	1. Be prepared for postural hypotension—responds to supine or Trendelenberg position 2. Nausea and vomiting may occur after rapid injection
Cimetidine (Tagamet)	Inhibits gastric acid secretion	300 mg q6h	May be diluted in 20 ml and given IV push over 1–2 min or mixed in 100 ml NS and infused over 15–20 min	1. Do not dilute with sterile water for injection
Dexamethasone (Decadron)	Corticosteroid used in the treatment of cerebral edema	IV–10 mg	4 mg/ml	1. Gradually reduce dosage on long term therapy 2. May mask or exacerbate infections 3. May cause GI ulceration or bleeding

Drug	Indications and Primary Effects	Dose	Preparation	Special Considerations
Diazepam (Valium)	Induces calming effects in anxiety disorders Anticonvulsant–used in the treatment of seizures	5–10 mg slow IV push (smaller doses indicated for elderly or debilitated patients)	5 mg/ml	1. Give slow IV push at 1 mg/min 2. Monitor respirations carefully 3. Do not mix with other IV drugs, flush with normal saline between doses
Digoxin (Lanoxin)	Increases the force of contractions and decreases the heart rate Used to treat atrial fibrillation and flutter, PATs, supraventricular tachycardia, and CHF	0.125–0.5 mg IV push	0.5 mg/2 ml	1. Administering calcium is contraindicated 2. Always check an apical pulse rate for 60 seconds prior to dose administration 3. Dosage should be given according to the patient's clinical condition
Diphenhydramine (Benadryl)	Antihistamine with anticholinergic effects Used to treat anaphylaxis, dystonic reactions, provide sedation	10–50 mg IV push	50 mg/ml	1. Used with epinephrine in anaphylaxis 2. If discharged after administration, caution against driving 3. Contraindicated in acute asthma attack
Dopamine (Intropin)	Indicated in hypertension Increased renal and mesenteric blood flow Increased heart rate and contractility–some vasoconstriction	Less than 5 μg/kg/min 5–20 μg/kg/min	800 mg in 500 ml D5W	1. Monitor vital signs and urine output closely 2. Incompatible with alkaline solutions 3. Watch for ventricular dysrhythmias and

Drug	Indications and Primary Effects	Dose	Preparation	Special Considerations
Dopamine (continued)	Vasoconstriction–decreased renal and mesenteric blood flow	Over 20 μg/kg/min		tachycardias 4. Titrate dosage according to blood pressure response
Epinephrine (Adrenalin)	Stimulates heart muscle and strengthens myocardial contraction Indicated for temporary relief of bronchospasm, treatment of anaphylaxis and asystole	0.5–1 mg (1:10,000) IV push IV infusion 1–8μg/min	1 mg/10 ml 2 mg in 500 ml D5W	1. If no IV exists, may be given into an endotracheal tube in cardiac arrest 2. Action of drug impaired if patient is acidotic, should be corrected prior to administration 3. May cause chest pain, dysrhythmias, tachycardia
Furosemide (Lasix)	Loop diuretic–used in treatment of pulmonary edema, hypertensive crisis, acute renal failure	40–200 mg	20 mg/ml	1. Give over 1–2 min for doses over 100 mg, push at 10 mg/min to prevent ototoxicity 2. Monitor blood pressure and pulse during rapid diuresis 3. May cause electrolyte imbalances especially potassium depletion
Heparin	Anticoagulant–inhibits clot formation in blood Used in treatment of thrombosis	Initial dose: 5,000 units by IV push Continuous infusion: 20,000–40,000 units/day	5,000 units ml 20,000–40,000 units/1,000 ml NS	1. Contraindicated in patients with bleeding disorders 2. Hemorrhage is the most serious complication. Observe for hematuria, bleeding gums, or black tarry stools.

Drug	Indications and Primary Effects	Dose	Preparation	Special Considerations
Hydralaz ne (Apresoline)	Peripheral vasodilator (lowers blood pressure)	10–20 mg	20 mg/ml	1. Dosage may be repeated as necessary 2. Myocardial stimulation may precipitate angina or myocardial infarction 3. Monitor blood pressure closely
Insulin	Antidiabetic agent– supplies insulin when natural producing source is deficient	Dosage according to bloodwork. (10–50 units usually administered with severe hyperglycemia)	100 units/ml	1. Monitor serum glucose 2. Observe for signs of hypoglycemia 3. Double check dose, insulin type, and expiration date with another nurse prior to administering
Isoproterenol (Isuprel)	Beta stimulator-increases contractility, heart rate Vasodilator Used as temporary measure until pacemaker insertion	2-20 μg/kg/min	2–5 mg in 500 ml D5W	1. Use at lowest dose possible to obtain a clinical response 2. Increases myocardial oxygen demand 3. May cause ventricular fibrillation or ventricular tachycardia 4. May cause hyperglycemia, nervousness
Lidocaine (Xylocaine)	Supresses ventricular dysrhythmias	Give 1 mg/kg bolus then 1–4 mg/min continuous infusion	2 g in 500 ml D5W (4 mg/ml)	1. Monitor for side effects: slurred speech, confusion, changes in level of consciousness

Drug	Indications and Primary Effects	Dose	Preparation	Special Considerations
Mannitol (Osmitrol)	Osmostic diuretic indicated for reduction of increased intracranial pressure	25–50 g	15%, 20%, 25% solution/ 500 ml over 30–60 min	1. Contraindicated in oliguria, so monitor output 2. Effects of drug begin within 15 min, but a rebound increase in intracranial pressure may occur after 12 hr 3. Vital signs must be monitored closely 4. Solution often crystalizes and may need to be warmed prior to infusion
Meperidine HCl (Demerol)	Narcotic analgesic– relieves pain without loss of consciousness	25–50 mg	50 mg/ml	1. May cause respiratory depression and hypotension especially if given too rapidly 2. Drug may mask symptoms so diagnosis should be made first 3. Hold medication if respirations are lower than 12/min
Metaraminol (Aramine)	Sympathomimetic indicated in hypotension—elevates systolic and diastolic blood pressure	15–100 mg	Dilute in 500 ml D5W or NS	1. Titrate infusion rate according to blood pressure 2. Will not replace blood or volume in the treatment of hypovolemic shock 3. Monitor blood pressure, pulse rate, urine output, color and temperature of extremities

Drug	Indications and Primary Effects	Dose	Preparation	Special Considerations
Methyl-prednisolone (Solu-Medrol)	Adrenocortical steroid potent anti-inflammatory agent Used in severe inflammation or immunosupression, also used in shock	10–250 mg	125 mg, 1 g	1. Administer slow IV push over 1 min or diluted in 100 ml IV fluid 2. Contraindicated in systemic infections 3. May mask or exacerbate infections
Morphine	Narcotic analgesic Indicated for pain in myocardial infarction, treatment of pulmonary edema, relief of dyspnea in acute left ventricular failure	5–15 mg	10 mg/ml	1. May cause respiratory depression, hypotension 2. Must be given slow IV push over 45 min 3. Use with caution in neurologic patients, as intracranial pressure may increase
Naloxone (Narcan)	Narcotic antagonist used to prevent or reduce effects of narcotic depression	0.4–2 mg IV push	0.4 mg/ml Infusion: 2 mg in 500 ml D5W	1. Dosage may be repeated or continuous infusion started if needed as effects of naloxone may be shorter than the narcotic
Nitroglycerin	Venous vasodilator, arterial vasodilator. At higher doses increases collateral coronary artery blood flow	No set dose—start at 5 μg/min and titrate to desired clinical effect	16 mg in 250 ml D5W (1μg/ml)	1. Use glass bottle and special tubing 2. Monitor blood pressure closely 3. Observe for headache, orthostatic hypotension
Nitroprusside (Nipride)	Arterial and venous vasodilator. Lowers blood pressure and preload	0.4 to 5.0 μg/kg/min	100 mg in 500 ml D5W	1. Light sensitive–cover infusion bag 2. Titrate dose to blood pressure response 3. Monitor blood pressure closely

Drug	Indications and Primary Effects	Dose	Preparation	Special Considerations
Norepi-nephrine (Levophed)	Alpha stimulator, vaso-constriction decreases renal blood flow. Used in patients with hypotension who are vasodilated	0.5–1.0 µg/kg/min titrated for effect	16 mg in 500 ml D5W	1. Monitor vital signs closely 2. If not infused in a Dextrose solution, potency is decreased 3. Tissue injury if extravasation occurs—may add 10 mg Regitine to infusion 4. May cause metabolic acidosis or dysrhythmias
Phenytoin (Dilantin)	Anticonvulsant–used in the treatment of grand mal and psychomotor seizures May also be used in ventri-cular arrhythmias unresponsive to lidocaine or procainamide	Initial loading dose 1 g	500 mg/10 ml	1. Must be given slow IV push at 50 mg/min 2. Cardiac arrest can occur if pushed too quickly 3. Should not be added to IV bag due to lack of solubility
Procainamide (Pronestyl)	Antiarrhythmic used to treat atrial fibrillation, paroxysmal atrial tachycardia, and ventricular tachycardia	Initial dose 100 mg q5min then 1–4 mg/min continuous infusion	2 g in 500 ml D5W	1. Run infusion at 20 mg/min until reach 1 g, desired effect, or side effects begin—widened QRS by 50% or hypotension 2. Maintenance drip to 1–4 mg/min 3. ECG should be monitored continuously–heartblock or cardiac arrest may occur 4. Must be administered cautiously in a person with myocardial infarction

Drug	Indications and Primary Effects	Dose	Preparation	Special Considerations
Trimethaphan (Arfonad)	Ganglionic blocker and vasodilator. Used in hypertension and cardiogenic shock	0.3–6 mg/min	500 mg (10 ml) in 500 ml of D5W	1. Keep patient supine to prevent cerebral hypoxia 2. Monitor for tachycardias and ventricular dysrhythmias 3. May cause local tissue extravasation 4. Incompatible with alkaline solutions
Vasopressin (Pitressin)	Vasoconstriction–causes smooth muscle contraction of the GI tract; used in acute GI bleeds	0.2–0.6 units/min	200 units in 500 ml NS or D5W	1. Monitor blood pressure and urine output closely 2. Check peripheral pulses and watch for signs of severe peripheral vasoconstriction 3. May cause dysrhythmias and hypotension

SUGGESTED READING

Bailey R, et al. Nurse's guide to drugs. Nursing 79. Horsham, PA: Intermed Communications, 1979:244.

Bernhart ER. Physicians's desk reference. Oradell, NJ: Medical Economics, 1987.

McIntyre KM. Cardiovascular pharmacology: part II. Manual for advanced cardiac life support. Dallas: American Heart Association, 1983:115.

White RD. Cardiovascular pharmacology: part I. Manual for advanced cardiac life support. Dallas: American Heart Association, 1983: 99.

E

LABORATORY TESTS

MARY E. MANCINI

Table 1 Reference Values for Therapeutic Drugs

Drug	Values
Acetaminophen	0–30 μg/ml
Amitriptyline + Nortriptyline	80–220 ng–ml
Nortriptyline	50–150 ng/ml
Amoxapine + 80H Amoxapine	200–500 ng/ml
Carbamazepine	4–12 μg/ml
Cyanide	0–0.05 mg/L
Thiocyanide	0–150.0 mg/L
Desipramine	150–300 ng/ml
Despiramine + Imipramine	150–250 ng/ml
Digoxin	0.8 –2.1 ng/ml
Doxepin + Desmethyldoxepin	150–250 ng/ml
Diazepam	0–1.0 mg/L
Lithium	1.0–1.6 mEq/L
Maprotiline	200–600 ng/ml
Phenobarbital	15–40 μg/ml
Phenytoin	10–20 μg/ml
Phenytoin, Free	1–2 μg/ml
Primidone	5–12 μg/ml
Procainamide	4–8 μg/ml
Protriptyline	76–260 ng/ml
Quinidine	2–5 μg/ml
Salicylate	< 20 mg/dl
Theophylline	10–20 μg/ml
Valproic Acid	50–100 μg/ml

Table 2   Reference Values for Cerebrospinal (CSF) Fluids

Product	Values
Cell count	
RBC	0
WBC	
Adult	0–10 lymphocytes/mm^3
Child	(>4 yrs) 0–20 lymphocytes/mm^3
Infant	(<1 yr) 0–30 lymphocytes/mm^3
Chloride	120–130 mEq/L
Glucose	40–70 mg/dl
MBP (myeline basic protein)	0–4 ng/ml
Protein	
Adult	15–45 mg/dl
Neonate	20–150 mg/dl
30–90 days	20–100 mg/dl
3–6 mo	15–50 mg/dl
6 mo–10 yr	10–30 mg/dl
Albumin	13.4–23.7 mg/dl
1gG	0.5–6.1 mg/dl
1gG/Albumin ration	0.08–0.14 mg/dl
1gG Index	0.34–0.58 mg/dl
1gG Synthetic rate	<3.3 mg/day

Table 3   Reference Values for Blood Specimens

Product	Value
Albumin	
Adults	3.9–5.0 g/dl
Infants	2.5–5.0 g/dl
Aldosterone	
Supine	5–20 ng/dl
Upright	10–34 ng/dl
Alkaline Phosphatase	
0–2 yr	80–270 U/L
2–5 yr	80–220 U/L
5–8 yr	60–230 U/L
8–12 yr	60–280 U/L
12–14 yr	60–320 U/L
14–16 yr	30–250 U/L
Adult	43–122 U/L
Amylase	30–110 U/L

Table 3   Reference Values for Blood Specimens (Cont'd)

Product	Value
Bilirubin, direct	< 0.3 mg/dl
Bilirubin, total	
Adult	< 1.3 mg/dl
Cord blood	< 3.0 mg/dl
24 hr	< 6.0 mg/dl
48 hr	< 10.0 mg/dl
Blood gases	
Arterial blood	
pH Adults	7.34–7.44
Infants	7.30–7.40
Po_2 Adults	75–100 mm Hg
Infants	60–90 mm Hg
Pco_2	35–45 mm Hg
HCO_3	22–26 mmol/L
Base	$- 2.4 - + 2.3$ mmol/L
O_2 cont	18–22 ml/dl
O_2 sat	95–98%
Hb CO	0–5%
Hb Met	0–1%
Venous blood	
pH	7.31–7.41
Pco_2	42–55 mm Hg
Pco_2	30–50 mm Hg
HCO_3	24–28 mmol/L
Base	$- 2.4 - + 2.3$ mmol/L
O_2 sat	60–80%
Calcium (total)	
Adults	9.1–10.6 mg/dl
Infants	8.5–10.0 mg/dl
Carbon dioxide (CO_2 content)	
Adults	22–31 mEq/L
Infant	22–26 mEq/L
CBC (automated hemogram)	
WBC	
Adults	$4.1–10.9 \times 10^9$/L
Newborn	$9.0–30.0 \times 10^9$/L
RBC	
Male	$4.3–6.2 \times 10^6$/mm³
Female	$3.8–5.5 \times 10^6$/mm³
Newborn	$4.4–5.8 \times 10^6$/mm³
Infant or child	$3.8–5.5 \times 10^6$/mm³
Hematocrit	
Male	40–52%
Female	37–46%
Newborn	53–65%
Infant	30–40%
Child	31–43%

Table 3 Reference Values for Blood Specimens (Cont'd)

Product	Value
Hemoglobin	
Male	13.2–16.2 g/dl
Female	12.0–15.2 g/dl
Newborn	15.0–22.0 g/dl
Infant	10.0–15.0 g/dl
Child	11.0–16.0 g/dl
MCV	
Male	2–105 μ^3
Female	79–101 μ^3
Newborn	96–108 μ^3
MCHC	
Male or female	31–34%
Newborn	32–33%
Platelet count	
Male or female	140–450 × 10^3/mm^3
Premature	100 – 300 × 10^3/mm^3
Leukocyte differential count	
Adults	
Segmented neutrophils	30–70%
Band neutrophils	0–10%
Lymphocytes	20–50%
Monocytes	2–12%
Eosinophils	0–7%
Basophils	0.2%
Chloride	
Adults	101–111 mEq/L
Infants	94–100 mEq/L
Cholesterol	107–307 mg/dl
Cortisol	10–25 μg/dl
CPK (creatinine phosphokinase)	
Male	57–374 U/L
Female	35–230 U/L
CK - MB	Negative
CK - MB%	0
Creatinine	
Adult	0.5–1.4 mg/dl
Infant	<1.0 mg/dl
Fibrin split products	<8 μg/ml
Fibrinogen	170–420 mg/dl
Folate (folic acid)	
Serum	>1.8 ng/ml
Free thyroxine index	4.5–11.5
Gastric	>90 pg/ml
Glucose	
Adults	65–110 mg/dl
Infants	40–110 mg/dl
Insulin	<20 μU/ml

Table 3   Reference Values for Blood Specimens (Cont'd)

Product	*Value*
Iron (total serum iron) (TSI)	
Male	55–140 μg/dl
Female	30–125 μg/dl
Iron binding capacity (TIBC)	
Male	253–415 μg/dl
Female	249–409 μg/dl
LDH (Lactate dehydrogenase)	
Adult	100–225 mU/ml
LDH–1	<85 IU
LDH–1/LDH	<35%
Potassium	
Adults	3.6–5.0 mEq/L
Infants	3.0–5.5 mEq/L
Protein	
Premature infants	4–6 g/dl
Term infant	5–7 g/dl
Adults	6–8 g/dl
Reticulocyte count	
Adults	0.5–1.5%
Newborn	1.1–4.5%
Infants	0.5–3.1%
Rheumatoid factor	<60 IU/ml
Sodium	137–145 mEq/L
Triglyceride	70–170 mg/dl
Urea nitrogen	
Adult	7–21 mg/dl
Infants	10–20 mg/dl
Uric acid	
Male	3.5–8.5 mg/dl
Female	2.5–7.5 mg/dl

Table 4 Reference Values for Urine Specimens

Product	Values
Amylase	<640 IU/L Random
Bile	Negative
Metanephrine	<1.3 mg/24 hrs
	<1.0 μg/mg Creat Random
Osmolality	
Males	392–1,090 mOsm/kg Random
Female	301–1,093 mOsm/kg Random
Urinalysis (UA)(adult)	
Specific gravity	1.002–1.030
pH	5–7
Protein	Negative
Glucose	Negative
Ketone	Negative
Bilirubin	Negative
Blood	Negative
RBC	0.3/hpl
WBC	0–5
Epl	0–1

SUGGESTED READING

Brater DC. Pocket manual of drug use in clinical medicine. 3rd ed. Toronto: BC Decker, 1987.

Brunner LS, Suddarth DS. The Lippincott manual of nursing practice. 3rd ed. Philadelphia: JB Lippincott, 1982:1467.

The Parkland Memorial Hospital Laboratory Manual. Dallas: Parkland Memorial Hospital, 1987.

NOTES

NOTES

NOTES